# Ocular Pharmacology and Therapeutics

*Acquisitions editor*: Caroline Makepeace
*Development editor*: Myriam Brearley
*Production controller*: Chris Jarvis
*Desk editor*: Claire Hutchins
*Cover designer*: Alan Studholme

# OCULAR PHARMACOLOGY AND THERAPEUTICS:

## A PRIMARY CARE GUIDE

**Michael J. Doughty**

PhD
Professor
Department of Vision Sciences
Glasgow Caledonian University
Glasgow
United Kingdom

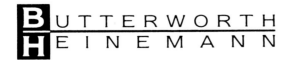

OXFORD AUCKLAND BOSTON JOHANNESBURG MELBOURNE NEW DELHI

Butterworth-Heinemann
Linacre House, Jordan Hill, Oxford OX2 8DP
225 Wildwood Avenue, Woburn, MA 01801-2041
A division of Reed Educational and Professional Publishing Ltd

ℛ A member of the Reed Elsevier plc group

First published 2001

Original material © DOCET (Directorate of Optometric Continuing Education and Training) 1997
Revisions and new material © Reed Educational and Professional Publishing Ltd 2001

**British Library Cataloguing in Publication Data**
A catalogue record for this book is available from the British Library

**Library of Congress Cataloguing in Publication Data**
A catalogue record for this book is available from the Library of Congress

ISBN 0 7506 4520 2

Typeset by David Gregson Associates, Beccles, Suffolk
Printed and bound in Spain

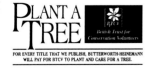

FOR EVERY TITLE THAT WE PUBLISH, BUTTERWORTH-HEINEMANN
WILL PAY FOR BTCV TO PLANT AND CARE FOR A TREE.

# Contents

# Foreword

The idea for this book was a result of the enthusiasm shown by UK optometrists for a series of articles published between 1997 and 1999. The modules, entitled *Ocular Pharmacology and Therapeutics*, were a huge success and saw record numbers of candidates responding to each individual assessment test. The series was funded by the Directorate of Continuing Education and Training (DOCET) and published and distributed by the journal *Optician*.

The thirst for knowledge of optometrists to gain more information about the investigation, diagnosis, and therapeutic management of ocular disease should be of no surprise to anyone. Yet Professor Doughty was surprised at the level at which practitioners wanted to increase their knowledge base. This book, which carries the same title as the earlier series of articles, represents a testimony to this. *Ocular Pharmacology and Therapeutics* is novel in that it not only covers each of the areas mentioned above, but it also probes the anatomical, physiological and pharmacological principles that are pertinent to the use of not only therapeutic pharmacological agents, but also to diagnostic pharmacological agents.

It is perhaps easily forgotten that the eye is not a passive cul-de-sac but an avenue for systemically-administered drugs to enter from the systemic circulation, and potentially cause some marked side effects. The optometrist is in a privileged position to assess such effects as tissues of the eye may show signs of an adverse drug reaction (ADR) to a systemic agent. It is with the latter in mind that two whole chapters, 5 and 7, representing one fifth of this book, are dedicated to this important area of medication-related adverse drug reactions. Just as importantly, the topical ocular administration of drugs can cause systemic ADRs and these are appropriately discussed as well.

There are many myths and fallacies concerning the role of ophthalmic corticosteroids in inflammation. Chapter 9 is dedicated to this area and aims to give an authoritative view, which it is hoped will go some way to allaying practitioner fears and dispelling some of the inaccuracies. The book concludes with a definitive chapter on the therapeutic management of arguably one of the most common conditions encountered by the optometric practitioner, namely primary open-angle glaucoma.

I hope that this book will be seen not only as a reference guide for the practitioner practising (or wishing to) ocular therapeutics but also as a useful manual that can be utilised in routine clinical practice. For those practitioners keen to keep abreast of new developments in ocular therapeutics, the reader is referred to another of the author's publications – *Drugs, Medications and the Eye*. Professor Doughty is also responsible for producing and maintaining an up-to-date drugs and ocular therapeutics database hosted at: www. academy. org and coming soon on www. optometryonline.net.

*Sandip Doshi*
*Clinical Editor*
*Optician*

## Acknowledgements

The publishers and the College of Optometrists, UK would like to thank Allergan for the sponsorship of the original supplements published in *Optician*. The author is indebted to the Directorate of Continuing Education and Training (DOCET) and the *Optician* for their support throughout this project

# An introduction: The issues surrounding the future expansion of optometrists' role in ocular therapeutics in the UK

## Therapeutics CET series

In 1997 the UK-based Directorate of Optometric Continuing Education and Training, with Optician, published a modular distance-learning course in ocular therapeutics and pharmacology. From January 1999, the course was published in 10 modules as bi-monthly supplements to Optician. Each module included multiple-choice questions, answers to be forwarded to DOCET for marking. This book is the overall outcome of this course, with some modifications and extra summary material.

## Introduction

Optometrists in the UK have been interested in an expansion of the scope of their practice for several years. They have demonstrated their interest by record attendances at a range of continuing education lectures offered by regional optometric associations, often under DOCET (Directorate of Optometric Continuing Education and Training) sponsorship.

The College of Optometrists made decisions in 1996 that should allow it to adopt

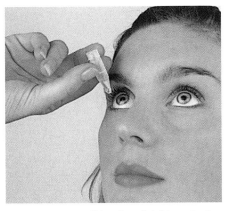

*Optometric prescribing: beneficial to patients and cost-effective, according to the NHS perspective.*

a more central role in ensuring that UK optometrists are fully trained and prepared for the management of ocular disease and use of ocular therapeutics in practice.[1] One College option has been the development of a syllabus for a higher diploma examination in therapeutics, and this syllabus was completed in 1998.[1]

Another option was to make a commitment, with support and financial backing from the opthalmic pharmaceuticals industry, to providing optometrists in the UK with distance-learning training on ocular therapeutics.

That the College chose such an option no doubt raised a few eyebrows, even though it was well in line with the then current NHS perspectives[2] and those of the British Medical Association. The latter is on record as stating: 'There is a real need for a wide breadth of knowledge to make the initial diagnosis and manage the condition.'[3]

Some have argued that this wide breath of knowledge can be achieved with formal continuing education for optometrists. Indeed, with another lobby group – The Patient's Association – stating that pharmacists should be given an expanded role in the primary care area,[4] this would also be achieved through pharmacists' widely-used continuing education programmes. Such MCQ-based evaluation procedures have also been used effectively in optometry for years.

It is widely accepted that the expanded scope of practice and understanding of how to treat eye disease requires a knowledge of the disease process and of the diagnoses,[5] yet the Royal College of

Ophthalmologists has insisted that eye disease treatment should only be carried out by medically trained doctors.[6] However, in an *ad hoc* survey of ophthalmologists, half agreed that optometrists, with suitable training, should be allowed to manage selected eye diseases.[7]

Furthermore, since the current NHS perspective is that 'with appropriate safeguards, it would be beneficial to patients and cost effective to extend the range of items that optometrists can prescribe', it behoves optometry not only to respond but also to prepare itself accordingly to meet all reasonable 'safeguards'. Similarly, just as recently the NHS Executive seems to have done, it is timely to note that the enormous and rapid change in the scope of practice achieved by US optometrists was based on a perspective by physicians and directors of university-based health care clinics that 'You don't need 10 years of training, four years at medical school, and six years of residency to deal with common visual problems.'[8]

The Opticians Act, 1989, required optometrists to refer all patients with abnormal conditions to their GP, without diagnosis[9] (New guidelines (Statutory Instruments 1999, No. 3267, OPTICIANS) introduced in January 2000 allow for changes to be made, including the recognition that UK optometrists can make a diagnosis).[32] Notwithstanding, what must be noted, is that it has been many years since the original protocols were established and the quality of optometric education and clinical abilities have improved considerably over the years.[9] The variation in the quality of the pre-registration year is, however, an issue for students and still needs to be tackled.[10]

Just as others have also noted, it is up to the profession, educators in charge of teaching and the registration body to determine the minimum teaching syllabus to produce a competent practitioner at an entry level standard,[11] with this standard now being primary eye care.

UK optometrists are in a position to respond to US thinking that long ago appreciated that if ophthalmology had addressed the public's total visual needs in the late 1800s – instead of the more limited scope of eye disease – the profession of optometry most likely would never have been born.[12] To follow the US example, 'Health plans do encourage primary care physicians to provide a broad scope of diagnostic and treatment services at the entry level.'[13] This initial entry point, or primary care, is the location where a patient enters the health care delivery system, or has access to health care.[13]

So, one might ask how this expansion of primary care can be achieved. Optometrists in the US recognised that the introduction of therapeutic drugs into optometric practice could only be achieved by gaining the confidence of their fellow professionals.[14] This is very important for the UK since it has been noted that 'GPs and other members of the primary health care team need to be educated about the actual and potential services that are available through optometrists, since they do not understand the abilities and skills of optometrists.'[2]

Times have changed from the days when an individual, who for the first time desired a pair of health service spectacles, had to get a recommendation from a medical practitioner. Theoretically, the physician was supposed to determine whether the applicant's symptoms were caused by eye defects of by some physical condition that might necessitate medical treatment.[15] The links needed nowadays are to establish 'appropriate speedy referrals to secondary care'[2] which not only recognise that optometrists could play a pivotal role in the administration of primary eye care but also, with GPs, might become an effective part of the primary care team.

## Strong advocates

It should also be noted that some community pharmacists have been strong advocates of their role in the management of eye conditions deemed suitable for over the counter (OTC) treatment without the intervention of any other medical specialist.[16]

The Royal Pharmaceutical Society has recently stated that 'community pharmacists will increasingly work alongside GPs and nurses as part of the primary care team, helping with prescribing and

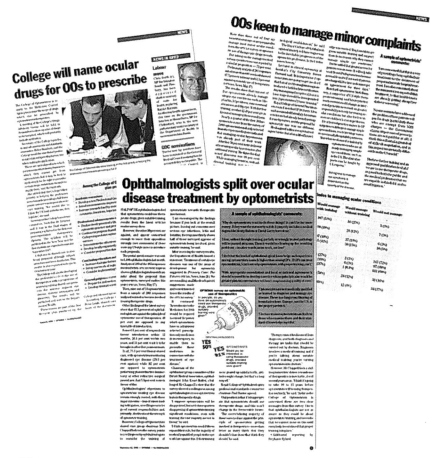

*Past debates on optometric use of therapeutics in the UK.*

medicines management.[17] Note the omission of optometrists in that statement.

Optometrists, according to current NHS perspectives, surely will also play a part in this primary care team by both providing diagnoses and treatment of eye disease, as well as increased use in management of medicines-related eye and vision problems. It should, however, be noted that registered pharmacists are required to keep abreast of pharmaceutical knowledge 'in order to maintain a high standard of professional competence'.[18] It is surely to be expected of UK optometrists that they also adopt far-reaching codes of ethics and practice through compulsory continuing education. The primary care perspective should include clinical examination and treatment procedures, ocular disease, ocular pharmacology and clinical medicine.[19]

Practitioners, as well as students, need to understand their responsibility in the treatment and management of eye disease as well as the potential for ocular and systemic complications to the use of medicines.[19] Such increasing responsibilities require there to be continuing education and training as a requirement for registration into the primary eye care domain.[14]

Since it may well be argued that not all practitioners may want to be involved in the expansion of their professional duties such as primary eye care including use of therapeutics, a subspecialty within the profession could develop.[11] What is important, therefore, is that all optometrists are encouraged to enhance their practices and advance their profession by expanding their range of responsibilities into primary eye care.[20]

Since it is likely that few US optometrists today would question the need for extended use of diagnostic and therapeutic pharmaceutical agents in a role as primary care providers,[12] training in the expanded use of such agents is a necessity. In addition, it should not be overlooked that an appropriate eye examination, accurate and reliable diagnosis and the treatment of all visual care needs is also part of this expanded scope of practice.[12] It is also essential to accept that the achievement of a pass at the entry (PQE) level to the profession does not fully prepare a person for their future career.[11]

Optometrists already working in a shared care environment are probably best-suited to treat a range of common ophthalmic conditions that do not require urgent

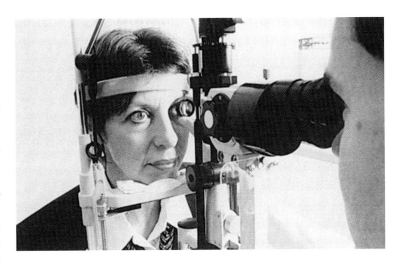

*Optometrists will need to be cognisant of diagnostic techniques.*

referral to a hospital.[9] Indeed, two-thirds of a sample of UK general practitioners responded to a survey by agreeing that optometrists should carry out treatment of external eye conditions such as conjunctivitis.[21] The UK optometrist should be able to take on the same roles as practitioners in the USA where those who treat eye disease can provide more comprehensive care at the primary entry level. Shared care schemes that use the full range of optometrists' skills can reduce the need for referrals to office-based and hospital-based physicians, including ophthalmologists.[13]

With the growth and ageing of the UK's population, the increased incidence and prevalence of eye diseases surely requires more accessible primary eye care, including the need for the more widespread use of therapeutics by all members of the primary care team.

While the drive to expand the scope of practice should not be solely justified by the higher prevalence of eye diseases,[22] optometrists should be able to define clearly conditions and diseases that are within the scope of optometric practice.[19] While concerns have been noted in the UK optical community and suggestions made that the treatment of corneal ulcers or glaucoma is beyond the scope of optometry,[23] this does not obviate the need to consider all eye diseases from the perspective of diagnoses.

Research by Crookes Health Care shows that the number of people suffering from minor eye complaints is on the increase, with the result that the OTC eye care market is now growing steadily.[24] The four most common diagnoses are bacterial conjunctivitis, allergic conjunctivitis, meibomian cyst and blepharitis.[25] Of the 8805 cases presenting to an accident and emergency department, 4.6% were eye-related, and 75.7% of these ocular cases were contact lens-related. Diagnoses deemed suitable for treatment by a contact lens practitioner were 43%.[26] As noted in the USA, for many inflammatory and infectious eye diseases, the initiation of early pharmaceutical therapy greatly improves the likelihood of effective treatment and lowers the risk of complications.[13]

## Aggressive screening

The burden on the higher levels of care appears to be so substantial that one hospital-based optometrist[27] noted that for those with severe eye disease, 'Unavoidably, many wait several months before being diagnosed by an ophthalmologist as having an often untreatable condition.' A more aggressive eye disease screening programme at the primary care level, in line with current NHS perspectives, would surely reduce the incidence of such secondary and tertiary care patients. Since the management of even common eye conditions requires a level of specialist knowledge and instrumentation that most GPs do not have,[20] optometrists could take the appropriate measures not only to respond to this need, but also to support fully other members of the primary health care team in the management of common eye diseases.

To do this, the high-street and hospital-based optometrist needs to be cognisant of the best and most recent diagnostic techniques, the differential diagnosis which need to be considered and the most appropriate treatments and management protocols.

With diagnoses being just as important as the ability to initiate appropriate therapeutic care and patient follow-up, a well-structured patient record should be the cornerstone of a primary care, problem-oriented optometric practice. The problem-oriented record, an unambiguous statement of clinical actions, encourages the optometrist to deal with patients' concerns, to think and act logically, and to provide appropriate and continuous care.[28]

An understanding of the required follow-up once therapeutic care has been initiated is just as important since appointments may well be missed simply because of difficulties in getting away from work or forgetfulness.[29]

It should be recognised that the initiation of primary therapeutic care requires that the optometrist be available for providing after care, or make every reasonable effort to ensure that a patient is advised of this in accordance with even current guidelines in the Opticians Act.

So, where does the pharmacology aspect of primary eye care fit in? Pharmacology is not the only course objective needed to prepare practioners or optometry students to provide competent therapeutic eye care,[19] but it is a vital component of the educational process.

Proper patient management requires far more knowledge and training than selection, route of administration, dosage, adverse reactions, costs and pharmacokinetic action of drugs. Pharmacology is just one component of the current continuing education process. These earlier perspectives have been consolidated both in further government and NHS initiatives,[30] and by the opinion of UK optometrists.[31] The 1999-published Crown Report,[30] further elaborates on the potential role of UK optometrists in primary eye care, while UK optometrists have unambiguously indicated their interest in primary eye care.[31] A practitioner-based survey,[31] sampling a reasonably wide spectrum of UK optometrists indicated significant support to management of anterior segment eye

disease. Within this context, the new referral guidelines[32] relating to diseases of the eye provide a logical mechanism by which UK optometrists can become involved in the management of non-sight-threatening eye disease.

# References

1 Bentley C (1996) College prepares ocular therapeutics examination. *Optometry Today* June 3, 14.

2 Nation Health Service (1996) *Primary Care: The Future*, p. 39.

3 Kist-Butler J (1996) Medics warn of eye drugs danger. *Optician* **211**: 7.

4 Howland G (1996) Patients back pharmacists. *Chemist Druggist* July 20, 78.

5 Hunter P (1996) Medics warn of eye drugs danger. *Optician* **211**: 7.

6 Anon (1996) Medics warn of eye drugs danger. *Optician* **211**: 7.

7 Anon (1996) Ophthalmologists split over disease treatment by optometrists. *Optician* **212**: 7.

8 Michigan Optometric Association (1989) Lobby Document 'What you should know about eye care . . . and the profession of optometry.

9 Kerr C (1996) Looking into high-street eye care. *Chemist Druggist* July 20, 90–91.

10 Editorial (1996) UMIST and UWCC plan registrable degrees. *Optometry Today* May 6, 14.

11 Vingrys AJ, Rumney NJ (1996) Optometric continuing education and training: The Australian experience. *Optometry Today* June 3, 21–24.

12 Ball RJ (1993) Whither goes our profession. *J Am Optom Assoc* **64**: 753–755.

13 Baresi BJ, Brooks RE (1994) Full-scope optometry meets managed care. *Optometric Economics* June, 10–13.

14 Alexander D (1996) The shape of things to come. *Optician* **211**: 17.

15 Lindsey A (1962) The Ophthalmic Service. In: *Socialized Medicine in England and Wales, The National Health Service 1948–1961.* The University of North Carolina Press, p. 426.

16 Clitherow J (1996) Seeing eye to eye with your patients. *Chemist Druggist/ Over the Counter* (suppl) May 25, 28–32.

17 Anon (1996) New-age visions for the future. *Chemist Druggist* Sept 14, 347.

18 Medicines, Ethics and Practice. A guide for Pharmacists (July, 1999). Royal Pharmaceutical Society of Great Britain **22**: 9.

19 Bartlett JD (1986) The didactic therapeutics curriculum. *J Optom Educat* **12**: 49–50.

20 Kerr C, Robertson G (1995) A matter of priority. *Optician* **209**: 18–19.

21 Agarawal R (1996) British Optometry: medical practitioners' opinion survey. *Br J Optom Dispensing* **4**: 50–53.

22 Soroka M (1986) The need for expanded scope of practice. *J Optom Educat* **12**: 46–48.

23 Shah RV (1996) *Optometry Today* May 20, 16.

24 Anon (1996) In the public eye. *Chemist Druggist* April 20, 94.

25 McDonnell PJ (1988) How do general practitioners manage eye disease in the community? *Br J Ophthalmol* **72**: 733–736.

26 Chatterjee AA, Bessant DAR, Naroo SA (1995) Ophthalmic accident and emergency department: Contact lens wearers. *Optometry Today* Nov 20, 23–25.

27 Rushen C (1996) Changes in hospital-based optometry. *Optometry Today* Feb 12, 33–36.

28 Baresi BJ (1984) Problem orientation. In: *Ocular Assessment: The Manual of Diagnosis for Office Practice.* Butterworth-Heinemann, pp. 3–10.

29 Mantyjarvi M (1994) No-show patients in an ophthalmological out-patient department. *Acta Ophthalmol* **72**: 284–289.

30 Department of Health (1999) *Review of Prescribing, Supply & Administration of Medicines. Final Report* (The Crown Report).

31 Doughty MJ, Rumney NK (1998) The future role of optometrists in the UK in treating anterior segment eye disease. *Optometry Today.* December 18, 33–37.

32 The General Optical Council (Rules relating to Injury or Disease of the Eye) Order of Council (1999). *Statutory Instruments 1999*, No. 3267.

# 1
# Legislation, legal aspects of medicine use and medicine types

Medicines legislation
Prescription writing and pharmaceutical abbreviations
Pharmaceutical labelling
Patient medications
Record keeping for patient medications
Routes of administration of medications
Fate of drugs in medications after administration

## Introduction

The diagnosis and management of ocular disease requires a reasonable understanding of the human body, rather than just considering the eye alone. Such activities could currently constitute the scope of practice of many different individuals who are directly or indirectly involved in the provision of health care, such as general medical practitioners, nurse practitioners, ophthalmologists and other medical specialists.

Optometrists in the UK have long enjoyed a status by which they are deemed capable of discriminating between normal and abnormal eye conditions such as to be able to arrange effectively for appropriate referral of patients to other health care professionals (Opticians Act, 1989, sections 26 and 31).[1] A long-standing part of this scope of practice has been the inclusion of the emergency management of eye disease (Opticians Act, 1989, section 31(5). With current amendments to the rules on referral relating to eye disease (and injury), the UK optometrist is deemed capable of making an actual diagnosis of an ocular condition, as opposed to just detecting an anomaly.[1]

As optometrists in the UK, supported by the College of Optometrists,[2] prepare for a more substantial role in the management of eye disease, it is appropriate to consider both the current status of optometric understanding of eye disease and its management, as well as what steps might be deemed necessary to develop further this understanding to encompass a wider scope of practice.

Given that local health care authorities can clearly categorise eye disease into several distinct types,[3] a logical mechanism is already in place to facilitate expansion of the scope of practice of UK optometrists. It is probably a given that, for the majority of practising optometrists in the UK, some reorganisation of their practice would be required for them effectively to assume the management of a wider spectrum of eye disease than undertaken now, even within emergency management guidelines.

Effective patient management is multifaceted and goes well beyond optometrists simply having knowledge of ocular therapeutic pharmaceutical agents (TPAs). Depending upon the new scope of practice that is ultimately realised, the optometrist nonetheless needs to consider current and future legislation for medicines (and the mechanism by which changes can be both effected and put into practice). Since access to medicines will be determined by optometrists collectively assuring the General Optical Council (GOC) and other regulatory agencies that they have the suitable training to be able to use, supply or prescribe a wider range of ophthalmic therapeutic drugs,[4] the goal of this chapter is to review the essential components of an understanding of medications, access to them and their use.

For any patient presenting with a manifest eye disease, the change in the comfort of their eye(s) or vision or the change in appearance of their eye(s) could be due to age, an endogenous systemic disease, or local eye disease. The medications a patient is taking always need to be considered since these can produce iatrogenic (caused by the process of medical examination or treatment) disease, or exacerbate a disease condition already present.

With the major contraindication to the use of any diagnostic or therapeutic pharmaceutical on the eye of a patient being a known allergy or sensitivity to the active drug or any other ingredient of the pharmaceutical, a comprehensive and accurate medical and medications record is essential to effective and safe practice. In some cases, a patient's past medication history can also be important.[5]

To be able to appropriately manage eye disease with medicines and to identify at-risk patients for any iatrogenic disease, the concurrent use of other ophthalmic pharmaceuticals or systemic medications needs to be considered to assess whether an enhanced or reduced response could occur to the planned pharmaceutical use. A complete medication record for a patient provides an extraordinarily useful insight into the patient's actual condition, rather than one having to rely simply on on-the-moment dialogue. To be able effectively to interpret the medication record of a patient, a knowledge of prescription writing, the reasons for selection of most different types of medications and the expected consequences of this selection need to be understood.

## Topical ophthalmic medications currently approved for optometric use

As designated by the Medicines Act and Opticians Act and their revisions (see below), the current pharmaceutical formulary available to optometrists encompasses a fairly wide spectrum of agents. Some of these are diagnostic pharmaceutical agents (DPAs) for professional use only by the optometrist on a patient, and are available through special access provisions even though they are designated as pre-scription-only medicines (POMs). Other therapeutic pharmaceutical agents have a P (pharmacy medicines) designation which permits use and supply, and others have a POM designation either for use and supply or use only.

Overall, these uses apply to some 35 listed drugs, although a number of these are essentially the same drug in terms of clinical use. Under special circumstances, optometrists may supply these drugs to their patients if the drug is identified as one for which there is a 'use and supply' designation or category, as opposed to a 'use only' designation. In such cases, patients can administer the pharmaceuticals to

themselves. This latter category includes consideration of the definition of emergency measures (see later).

Listed pharmaceuticals now approved for use and supply include those containing staining agents (fluorescein sodium ophthalmic solution, rose bengal ophthalmic solution), cholinergic blocking (antimuscarinic) mydriatic/cycloplegic eyedrops (tropicamide, atropine, cyclopentolate, homatropine, hyoscine), sympathomimetic mydriatics (phenylephrine eyedrops up to 10%), sympathomimetic decongestants/vasoconstrictors for topical ocular use (xylometazoline, naphazoline), direct and indirect-acting parasympathomimetic miotic eyedrops (pilocarpine, carbachol, physostigmine), antihistamines for topical ocular use (antazoline eyedrops up to 1%) and antimicrobial drugs for topical ophthalmic use (chloramphenicol eye drops up to 0.5%, chloramphenicol eye ointment up to 1%, propamidine eyedrops, dibromopropamidine eye ointment).[6]

There are other drugs listed in the formulary for which pharmaceuticals are not marketed, even as generics. These include low concentrations of adrenaline salts, ephedrine, bethanecol chloride, and neostigmine, mafenide and sulphacetamide sodium.

Within the context of use and supply, optometrists may administer pharmaceuticals containing the designated drugs to patients as part of their normal professional practice and also supply these pharmaceuticals to their patients on the condition that: 'The sale or supply shall only be in the course of their professional practice and only in an emergency'.

The use-only category includes drugs for topical ocular use in a professional capacity such as anaesthetic eyedrops (amethocaine, oxybuprocaine, proxymetacaine, lignocaine) and antibacterial drugs (framycetin eyedrops, framycetin eye ointment). As with the use-and-supply category, there are also listed drugs that are no longer available or marketed as pharmaceuticals, such as thymoxamine eyedrops and oxyphenbutazone ointment.

Optometrists may administer pharmaceuticals containing the drugs in the use-only category, but not supply these pharmaceuticals to a patient for self-use.

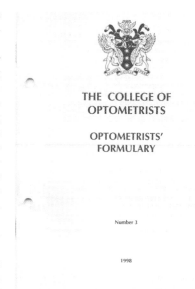

**Figure 1.1**
Optometrists' Formulary. (*Reproduced by kind permission of the College of Optometrists*).

## Sources of medicines information and regulations pertaining to optometric practice in the UK

Since the use of medicines is defined by law and optometrists only have access to designated medicines for use on the public, a review of the legalities of the availability and use of medicines is appropriate. These could be changed in several ways to facilitate the expanded scope of practice by optometrists.

The use of drugs by optometrists is determined by both the Opticians Act and the Medicines Act.[7] The Opticians Act, as updated in 1989 (section 31),[1] states that the GOC can make rules regulating the administration of 'drugs' by optometrists. These sorts of rules are contingent upon the provisions of the Medicines Act of 1968, as defined for optometrists in 1978, and with respect to several other modifications made between 1983 and 1989.

The two Acts, and their consequences, are periodically reviewed, especially by the College of Optometrists' Drug Advisory Panel (with optometrists represented). The main result is the preparation of the 'Optometrists' Formulary' by the College.[6] The formulary outlines which medicines can be legitimately used and supplied by optometrists within their normal scope of practice (Figure 1.1).

Before considering the types of changes in law that would need to be discussed before a practical expansion of the scope of optometric practice, it should be noted that optometrists, as well as orthoptists and dispensing opticians, may be involved in the observation of and/or provision of advice to their clients on the use of certain medicines that are generally available to the public. A comprehensive understanding of the Medicines Act and how it pertains to the eye is thus important.

The classification of drugs relevant to use by optometrists is covered specifically by the Medicines Act and is entirely consistent with the categorisation of medicines in the various pharmaceutical directories that are also available.

The Medicines Act was devised to make the process of drug (medicines) administration, supply and sale as easy, safe and uncomplicated as possible. Unless designated otherwise, current legislation dictates that all medicines be supplied by registered pharmacists.

There are exemptions, for example some medicines are listed on a general sale list (GSL) and are available from a range of retail outlets, while designated quantities of certain pharmaceuticals (drugs) can be supplied to an optometrist, with the approval of a registered pharmacist, on receipt of a signed order – that is, a written request on the optometrist's letterhead. These pharmaceuticals could be for diagnostic or therapeutic use.

Since the order and the resultant sale must stipulate the exact quantities of medicines required, the receiving optometrist is legally responsible for keeping records on the ultimate use of these medicines. Optometrists, depending on the stipulations of the sale, are allowed either to use these pharmaceuticals on their patients as appropriate and as part of an eye examination, or to administer the pharmaceuticals to their patients for management of certain emergencies.

Within the medicolegal context of such supply, detailed records of the use of exempted POM pharmaceuticals should be kept (Medicines Act 1968, section 112). It could be argued that detailed lists of the use of pharmaceuticals under the GSL or P categories do not need to be kept by an optometrist,[8] but details should clearly be included in a patient's records.

Therefore, in practical terms, records detailing the pharmacy stock and records of use and supply of individual items should be kept for all POM-designated pharmaceuticals.

Within strict guidelines, optometrists may also relabel prepackaged POM pharmaceuticals (preparations) specifically for patient use without holding a manufacturer's licence for assembly of pharmaceuticals. Under the provisions of the regulations for labelling of a 'dispensed medicinal product', the label must state the name of the patient (who must be physically present), the directions for use, the date of the supply and the name and address of the supplying optometrist. Other on-label details should include appropriate cautionary phrases such as 'For external use only', 'Not for consumption' or 'Keep out of reach of children'.

Pharmacy and GSL medicines, and presumably any non-medicines product intended for ocular use, should not be relabelled unless a specific approval and licence is granted to the individual optometrist.

## Classification of medicines – the details

The Medicines Act defines medicines by placing them in one of three main lists or categories. There is also a non-medicines list which includes ophthalmics. The designation is for pharmaceuticals or products, not drugs *per se* since a certain drug, as an ingredient of a branded (proprietary name) or generic named pharmaceutical, can be found in products designated under more than one category depending upon quantity of the drug in the pharmaceutical and its indicated use. The three medicines categories are:

• **The general sale list**, denoted by GSL and as defined by Section 51 of the Medicines Act and generally available for use by the public. The GSL designation of medicinal products can be taken to reflect the nature of the ingredients, the quantities or concentrations of the drugs in the pharmaceuticals and the designated end-use of these products. Within this context, GSL products are considered as safe, and unlikely to precipitate significant adverse reactions unless there is a specific sensitivity (allergy) to the drugs or other ingredients – thimerosal in contact lens care solutions as a cause of local and systemic allergy, for instance – or the product is

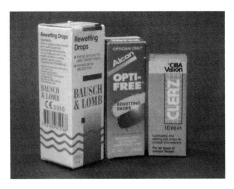

**Figure 1.2**
C€-marked, contact lens rewetting solutions.

abused – acetylsalicylic acid can cause ulceration of the alimentary tract if used excessively, especially in susceptible individuals.

The public can thus obtain these GSL medicines without supervision, and it is the end-user who then assumes responsibility for using the product as directed, reading and respecting any warnings or specific precautions about the use of these medicines and keeping them away from other potential users, such as children. GSL medicines are sometimes referred to as 'off-the-shelf'.

Among these products are contact lens care products including saline, cleaning and disinfecting solutions, other eye products such as sterile saline, as well a number of topical or systemically administered products for 'minor' medical ailments, for instance analgesics and alimentary tract remedies. Current legislation means that many contact lens-related products are marketed under a special category with the products carrying a C€ label. This includes most contact lens rewetting solutions (Figure 1.2).

An alternative method of placing non-contact lens-related ophthalmic products into the off-the-shelf category is by labelling them as a daily beauty care product or as cosmetic products. This category has long included various around-the-eye solutions, creams, powders, and pads for cleansing and/or beauty care, but also has included products such as lid cleansers (for blepharitis), eye salves and some lotions.

At the present time, the availability of any form of ophthalmic products (including contact lens care products) by mail order or via the Internet (www) is

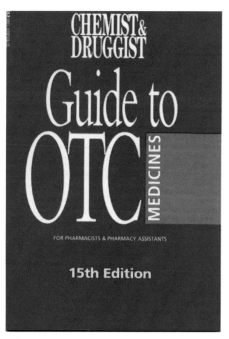

**Figure 1.3**
Guide to OTC Medicines. *Copies of the guide can be purchased from Miller Freeman UK Ltd.*[9]

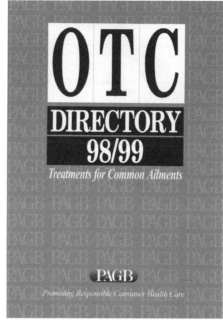

**Figure 1.4**
OTC Directory. *Copies of the guide can be obtained from the Proprietery Association of Great Britain.*[10]

**OTRIVINE-ANTISTIN** Ciba Vision
*Sympathomimetic/antihistamine.*
Xylometazoline hydrochlor. 0·05%, antazoline sulph. 0·5%; drops.
10 ml, £2·13 **(R)** £3·49.
**INDICATIONS:** Allergic conjunctivitis.
**ADULTS:** 1 or 2 drops two or three times daily.
**ELDERLY:** 1 drop two or three times daily.
**CHILDREN:** Under 5 years, not recommended; over 5 years, 1 drop two or three times daily.
**C/I:** Narrow angle glaucoma. Contact lenses.
**S/P:** Hypertension, hyperthyroidism, diabetes, coronary disease, dry eyes.
**INT:** Clonidine.
**ADR:** Transient stinging, headache, drowsiness, blurred vision. Rebound congestion.

**¶ LIVOSTIN** Ciba Vision
*Antihistamine.* Levocabastine (as hydrochlor.) 0·5 mg/ml; drops.
4 ml, £8·49.
**INDICATIONS:** Allergic conjunctivitis.
**ADULTS:** 1 drop per eye twice daily. Increase if necessary to three or four times daily; max. treatment period or use in any one year, 4 weeks.
**CHILDREN:** Under 9 years, not recommended; over 9 years, same as adult.
**C/I:** Renal impairment.
**S/P:** Pregnancy. Soft contact lenses.
**ADR:** Local irritation, blurred vision, oedema, urticaria, dyspnoea, headache.
▼ Report **any** adverse reaction to CSM.

**Figure 1.5**
*Pharmaceutical listings found in* MIMS *(see Figure 1.6)*

under review. A number of C€-labelled products are accessible by this route.

• **Pharmacy medicines**, denoted by P and as defined by Section 52 of the Medicines Act solely for supply through a retail pharmacy subject to some special exemptions. The term over-the-counter (OTC) medicines is widely used for such products. Directories are published that list these products under an OTC category, for instance, *Guide to OTC Medicines*[9] (Figure 1.3) or the *OTC Directory*[10] (Figure 1.4). All drugs on this list are generally sold or supplied from a registered pharmacy under the supervision of a registered pharmacist.

The P designation indicates that the ingredients, their concentrations and their indicated uses as medicines are such that they are generally safe for use by the public without medical supervision. However, their ingredients, the concentrations and their indicated uses are such that a control step for the supply is included so a professional can monitor their supply and make decisions on the suitability of the patient to use these products.

This control step largely relates to ensuring that certain warnings or pre-cautions will be provided to the end-user at the time of the sale. For instance, the pharmacist will be expected to ask several specific questions relating to the listed indications, contraindications (C/I), specific precautions (S/P), possible interactions (INT) and sometimes provide an additional warning on potential adverse drug reactions (ADRs). From an ocular perspective, these products include certain eyedrops for relief of irritated eyes, artificial tears, astringents and some eyewashes. For instance, the decongestant–antihistamine combination eyedrop P Otrivine–Antistine carries the C/I for narrow-angle glaucoma, listed S/Ps include high blood pressure, coronary disease, hyperthyroidism, diabetes and dry eyes, a listed drug interaction (INT) with the potent anti-high blood pressure drug clonidine, and listed ADRs of transient stinging and headache (Figure 1.5).

The P designation for medicines also includes a large number of other general remedies for allergies, alimentary tract disorders, skin irritation, personal hygiene and sleep disorders – all with a similar array of miscellaneous C/I, S/P, INT and ADR notes.

While the end-user assumes responsibility for the correct use of such products, the pharmacist or other health care professional assumes responsibility for providing the end-user with the appropriate instructions for use. Such instruction can be provided in a similar fashion to the instructions for use on writing a prescription for POMs (see below).

Rather than being off-the-shelf, these products will generally be supplied by the pharmacist on receipt of a specific verbal request from a consumer. Usually only single products will be sold under such a P designation – the availability of multiple products should be via a general medical practitioner or other appropriate professional person. When P medicines are used in the practice of a health care professional, or supplied to a patient from such a practice, the professional also assumes responsibility for instructing the patient on the use of the pharmaceutical.

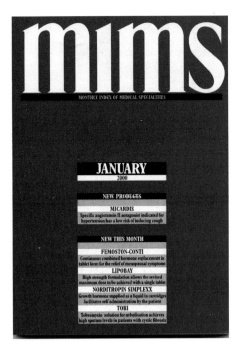

**Figure 1.6**
*A current copy of* MIMS (Monthly Index of Medical Specialities) *should be in every practice. MIMS (above) contains details of indications, contraindications (C/I), specific precautions (S/P), possible interactions (INT) and possible adverse drug reactions (ADR) for all prescription-only (POM; designated by the ¶ symbol) and most pharmacy (P) medicines. Text examples illustrated in Figure 1.5 are for (top) P Otrivine-Antistine, (bottom) POM Livostin. (With permission)*

- **Prescription only medicines**, denoted by POM and as defined by Section 58 of the Medicines Act. The current edition of *MIMS (Monthly Index of Medical Specialities)*[11] lists almost 2000 different brand pharmaceuticals (excluding vitamins, nutritional supplements, devices and hospital products), of which some 80% are POM-designated (Figure 1.6). There are also some 3000 generic products now on the market. A similar directory, the BNF (British National Formulary[12]), contains details of POM-designated products and a good indication of the availability of generic products (Figure 1.7).

Under current legislation, the POM term can be taken literally to mean that the designated pharmaceutical should only be available via prescription; prescription writing is also designated as being by doctors, dentists or veterinar-

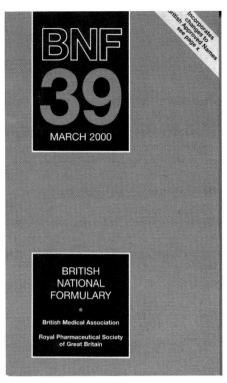

**Figure 1.7**
British National Formulary (BNF).

ians. The restricted access to POMs can be considered as a measure to ensure the safety of these medicines for use on or by the public. As a general guideline, POM listings designate those pharmaceuticals that contain drugs (or higher concentrations of drugs) for which there should be some supervision in their use. This 'supervision', or patient selection, is the responsibility – by literal interpretation of section 65 of the Medicines Act – of the health care provider who writes the prescription.

The rationale, from a drugs perspective, is that the risks of ADRs are generally higher for POM than for P or GSL products, with the key difference being the quantity of the drug in the pharmaceutical and thus the amount that might reasonably be taken as a single dose. While the number of limitations to use of POMs (i.e. the information listed under C/I, S/P, INT, and ADR) may not be substantial, it is the potential consequences of these limitations being ignored that has been considered.

The interpretation of these limitations is considered the realm of the health care specialist. So, for example, directory listings for the POM antihistamine

eyedrops containing levocabastine (POM Livostin) do not include narrow-angle glaucoma under C/I, although it might logically be considered as possible based on reports with first-generation oral antihistamines such as chlorpheniramine, but note that patients with renal impairment should not be prescribed this product. Similarly, caution is recommended for the use of these eyedrops in pregnancy (see Figure 1.5).

Both decisions on renal capacity and pregnancy are thus the realm of the general medical practitioner or equivalent, since less-than-expected rates of drug clearance from the body (bioelimination, see later) could lead to excess histamine $H_1$-blocking effects in the body while the effects on the fetus have probably not been determined in humans.

The listed ADRs for POM Livostin also include local irritation, blurred vision, oedema, urticaria, dyspnoea and headache. In a similar vein to the listed S/Ps, the diagnosis and management of the potential systemic complications (urticaria, dyspnoea and headache) are considered the realm of the doctor. However, unless there are extraordinary circumstances, the listed ADRs are generally no more substantial than for the P Otrivin–Antistin (see Figure 1.5) eyedrops containing the antihistamine and decongestant, and it could be argued that the precipitation of acute angle-closure through (excessive) use of P Otrivin–Antistin eyedrops in patients with narrow/closed anterior chamber angles could be more serious than local urticaria.

In the opinion of this writer, the idiosyncrasies among the C/I or S/P listings require just as much discernment and should provoke greater debate. An example here is the more recent C/I listings that include soft contact lenses, implying that the precipitation of a (mild) adverse reaction related to interaction of eyedrop preservatives with the corneal epithelium is of the same degree of severity as an angle-closure glaucoma (with real risk of blindness due to irreversible corneal endothelial damage), or systemic antihistamine overdose (presumably risking precipitating ventricular tachycardia), and of a higher risk than sympathomimetic ($H_1$-blocking) effects on fetal blood flow. This 'C/I' perspective on the use of eyedrops in contact lens wearers is however very much under review,[13] and some more recent ophthalmic products now carry a note of 'Do not use while or immediately before wearing contact lenses'.

Notwithstanding, it is the responsibility of the re-trained optometrist not only to be familiar with all these limitations to use of POMs, but also to be able to manage patients effectively and safely.

Under current legislation, special exemptions are extended to optometrists who may purchase a specific number of these prescription-only medicines for professional use. A signed order must be presented to a pharmacist on the optometrist's letterhead and it must be a request for the 'supply' of the designated pharmaceutical and the quantity required, i.e. $36 \times 5$ g tubes of Atropine Eye Ointment 1%.

UK optometrists have had access to several POM pharmaceuticals that are not only designated TPAs but which are intended for emergency management of bacterial eye infections or, prophylactically, to reduce the risk of an infection developing.[6]

Since the classification of medicines is regularly reviewed, pharmaceuticals that were once considered only for POM classification are now widely available as pharmacy medicines (e.g. POM Livostin and P Livostin Direct are currently marketed). The reason for such changes is simply that the more a drug or pharmaceutical is used by the public, the more the health care profession understands about the efficacy as well as the limits to the use of the drug or pharmaceutical. If the frequent use of a pharmaceutical produces no significant adverse reactions or drug–drug interactions, then there is no longer a good reason for retaining the POM designation.

The review process also imposes a stricter safety review when there is uncertainty about limitations in the use of a pharmaceutical. When a new pharmaceutical is released for prescription-only use, it will usually carry a specific note in the directories that the Committee on the Safety of Medicines (CSM) must be informed if any adverse reactions are encountered (see Figure 1.5). This requirement for reporting adverse drug reactions (ADRs) may stay in place for up to 2 years after the pharmaceutical or drug is released for POM use, depending on how much it is used.

## Prescription writing and pharmaceuticals-related abbreviations

Prescription writing is the specific request to a pharmacist to provide a named patient with a POM-designated pharmaceutical.[14] The prescription is written by an individual who is considered able to identify the patient as being suitable for the medication based on both the diagnosis of the patient's disease or ailment and on discerning that the patient is not at risk for serious complications (ADRs).

Using POM Livostin as an example again, guidelines in the example given state that the product is not recommended for use on children under the age of 9 years, but that the same dosage (up to four times daily) can be used for adults as well as children aged over 9. When risks are perceived, the patient may still be prescribed the medication but for use only under certain conditions. The prescription can therefore also contain specific instructions for the identification or use of the medicine that should take into account any precautions that are deemed necessary.

A prescription (on appropriate official forms) contains specific information deemed necessary safely and reliably to supply a patient with medication(s). The essence of such a form is illustrated in Figure 1.8; although the details differ slightly for different parts of the UK, especially on the reverse of the form. Such prescription form blanks are only available to licensed prescribers. As shown, a prescription, depending on its type, will generally contain information including the patient's name and address (initials and one full surname), the designated product inscription (i.e. the brand name and, where appropriate, the strength of the pharmaceutical), the subscription (i.e. volume of bottle to be dispensed, number of tablets, etc), the signatura (sometimes prefixed by the abbreviation Sig) which are the directions for use of the product that is to be given to the patient by the pharmacist. The writing of a prescription does not necessarily mean that it will be filled as written. A local authority and especially an NHS paid-prescription may be subject to local or regional rules, e.g. the Drug Tarrif, and/or automatic generic product substitution.

To the signatura, the pharmacist may also add any appropriate general instructions, such as 'for external use only', or 'not for internal use' for eyedrops. Checking the NP box (do not name the drug) is occasionally used in the hope of reducing patient confusion or anxiety about medications, and the pharmacist would just ensure that the product was labelled in general terms, for instance 'the tablets'.

The prescription form must be signed and dated by the doctor, who may also be identified in the box below the signature either as an individual or a hospital trust. Prescription pads also carry a designated numbered system to identify each prescriber. A superscription, i.e. a designation as to whether the product is prescription-only, will not usually be used simply because the product is unambiguously identified by its brand name or generic equivalents (see section below).

The date is important because, normally, a prescription should only be filled by a pharmacist within 6 months of its writing and only a designated number of times according to the written instructions they receive. Under special circumstances, a pharmacist may refill a prescription under emergency guidelines without written instructions, but on the understanding that written instruction will follow.[14]

## Medication information and patient records

Medication information is essential for the management of eye disease. Both to diagnose appropriately patients' diseases or ailments, and identify the suitability of a patient for treatment with a specific medication, details of concurrent medication use is essential. It is only through this knowledge that it is possible both to identify and appropriately respond to listed C/Is, S/Ps and potential drug interactions (INTs). Time needs to be assigned to taking such a medications and health history (Figure 1.9). Directories such as MIMS and BNF generally only list this information, but the *ABPI Compendium of Data Sheets*[15] contains much more information and some explanation of why these cautionary notes exist. This sort of information, and

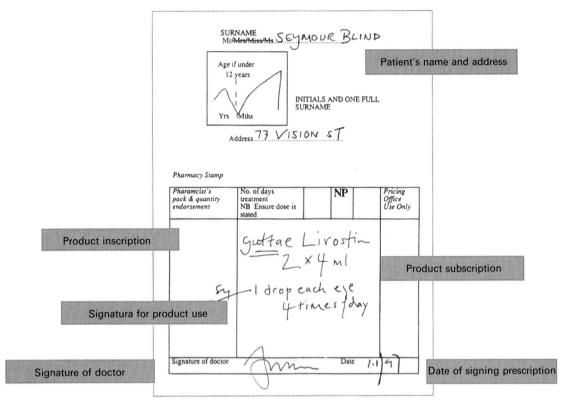

**Figure 1.8**
*The principal components of a prescription form for pharmaceuticals, as completed by the prescribing doctor, and to be presented to a licensed pharmacist. See text for explanation of terms.*

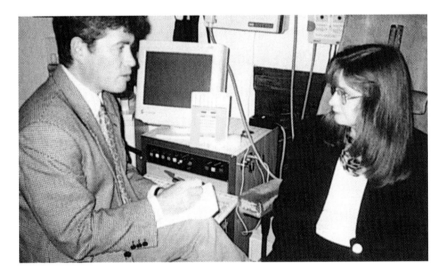

**Figure 1.9**
*Medication history. Both to diagnose appropriately a patient's disease or ailment and identify the suitability of a patient for treatment with a specific medication, details of concurrent medication use is essential.*

supporting explanation along with patient guidelines, can be found from a variety of sources, especially texts written for nurses.[16] As a practical working guideline, one should not expect a patient to volunteer this information.

Gathering the appropriate and correct information on a patient's medications, and about the way the patient is actually using them, is a prerequisite for responsible and safe practice. It is essential that the information collected is correct and informative and this can be easily achieved by paying attention to a few simple details.

Medications generally have a specific name. This is called a brand, branded, or proprietary name and this name is usually registered. For example POM Catapres is a brand-name product containing clonidine which is listed as a possible source of a drug–drug interaction for the use of P Otrivine–Antistin.

As another example, consider the listed interactions for oral acetazolamide (POM Diamox) which include 'folic acid antagonists' – a group of drugs represented by the sulphonamides. One current use of these is for ulcerative colitis, for which a branded product is POM Salazopyrin. However, there are also several generic pharmaceuticals available marketed by different companies. Such generic equivalents still have

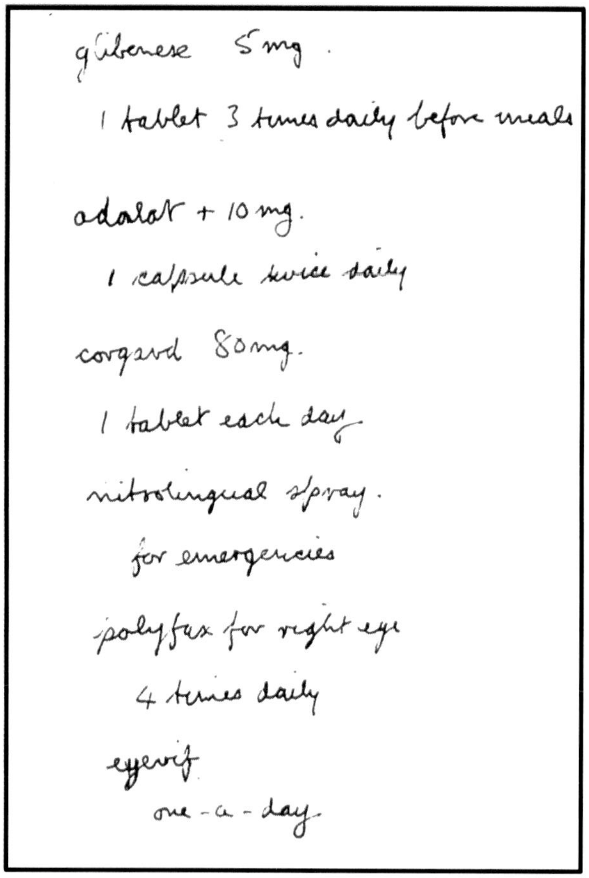

**Figure 1.10**
*A hand-written medications list provided by a patient to a practitioner. Further details of the brand-named products, except the vitamins, can be found in* MIMS *or a* BNF *by consulting the index.*

a name on the product but it identifies the drug (sulphasalazine) in the medicine and has a non-proprietary name (POM Sulphasalazine) which should be noted along with the company that produced it (i.e. POM Sulphasalazine, Cox Pharms). Such products may be also listed on an NHS-approved prescription service, in which case they can be identified to that source (NHS Sulphasalazine).

Information on the medications may be presented to a health care professional in several ways:

- **Verbally**. This method may be limited, incomplete and often in lay language, e.g. heart tablets, water pills, lots of aspirin, etc. In taking this information, it needs to be corrected and it is advisable to check for errors, for instance by consulting *MIMS* or a *BNF*, before using it for patient records or for referral letters etc.
- **As a hand-written list**. This is a preferred method to the verbal one. An example is illustrated in Figure 1.10. Medications will often be referred to by brand names, but perhaps without details of quantities and/or frequency of use. Try to get details of dosage, etc., especially if a patient is symptomatic.

## Goals for quality patient medication records

Assuming reasonable patient compliance with any recommendations for medication use, a full medication record is a useful insight into a patient's state of health and state of mind. If a patient is symptomatic or showing signs of drug–drug interactions (adverse effects), this information can be used in the diagnosis of their condition as well as in making appropriate plans, such as for a referral.

It is more than simply a good habit to check the identity and spelling of medications in a current *MIMS* or *BNF*, as errors could lead to disastrous consequences. It is bad practice to accept a 'medications same as last visit' for patient records, since the last records may not be available when needed and a patient's recall may be wrong.

It is also a good idea to indicate, on patients' records that appropriate questions have been asked about medications and allergies. If the answer to either question is no, the record should clearly state this. Some of the goals of collecting medication history data (Figure 1.11) are to find out:

- What medications a patient is taking, or has recently been taking – the medications preferably should be identified by brand name. Their main drug(s) ingredients can be later identified by generic names.
- Why the patient is taking these medications – this information provides an excellent opportunity to check for accuracy especially when medication use is communicated verbally.
- How much of these medications a patient is taking – the goal here is to get an idea of whether they are taking their medications at a low, medium, or high dose. A *MIMS* or *BNF* will provide the normal adult dosage.
- When these medications are being taken. This will assist in making a diagnosis, especially for symptomatic patients when a drug interaction is suspected.
- How long a patient has been taking these medications. This information is more important when progressive adverse drug reactions that affect the eye are being investigated.

Whenever there are any uncertainties, concerns or questions about the adequacy and/or safety of these medications by current perspectives, a patient can, and should be, referred back to the doctor who prescribed their medications. With a changed scope of practice, it would presumably be the optometrist who would be prepared to respond to equivalent queries from a general practitioner or another doctor.

## Goals for quality patient medication records

- What medications a patient is taking
- Why the patient is taking these medications
- How much of this medication is a patient taking
- When these medications are actually being taken
- How long a patient has been taking these medications

**Figure 1.11**
*Some simple suggestions for a systematic approach to obtaining details for patient medication records.*

## Medicine (pharmaceutical) administration to the human body

An appreciation of the normal and unexpected consequences of patient medications is best achieved through an understanding of why a particular pharmaceutical is used. This issue addresses the actual pharmaceutical dosage and not really the drug itself.

Both prescription and medication information should include details on how the drug is to be delivered to the body. Medications, i.e. pharmaceuticals, can be administered to the human body by many different methods – by mouth (po), eyedrops (gtt), topical skin products (creams) etc.

Most pharmaceuticals are manufactured and packaged in such a way so as to optimise their actions when administered in a particular mode.[17,18] This is the recommended method of administration, and health care practitioners should avoid using pharmaceutical products in a way that is not recommended. Regardless of the extent of current or future involvement in the management of eye disease, it is the optometrist's role to ensure there is an understanding of what patients should be doing with their medications, in terms of the administration of these medications, and be able to answer basic questions on different modes of administration.

An understanding of the administration of medicines should also alleviate uncertainties and ensure that appropriate 'language' is used. This information is of use for patients' records, and may also be needed when patients' medications records

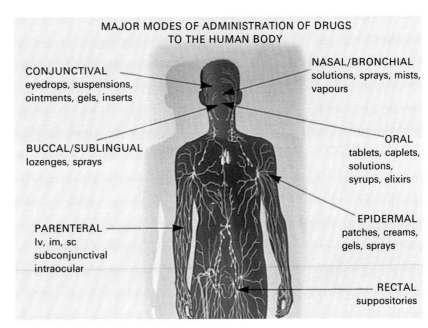

**Figure 1.12**
*Major modes of administration of drugs to the human body. A pharmaceutical type is selected to optimise delivery of the drug(s) it contains either to the whole body, or select internal or external parts of the body.*

are being communicated to another health care provider. In including such information in patients' records, or communicating this information to someone else, slang terminology should be avoided. For example, generally speaking, patients take or are administered 'medications' not 'drugs'.

The modes of administration of medicines are summarised in Figure 1.12 and discussed below.

- **Conjunctival administration.** This is the formal term for the route of entry of drugs from an ophthalmic pharmaceutical, across the corneal and conjunctival surfaces into the eye or the rest of the body. Ophthalmic pharmaceuticals can be in the form of solutions, suspensions, oils or liquid gels, all of which are instilled into the eye. It is likely that all will be referred to as 'guttae'. Alternatively, ophthalmic pharmaceuticals can be in the form of ointments or gels applied to the conjunctiva or to the lid margin, which are likely to be abbreviated as 'ung'.

  Lastly, there are some special modes of conjunctival delivery which take the form of wafers, inserts (Ocusert) or collagen shields, all of which are touched to, placed upon or inserted into the lower conjunctival sac. The pharmaceutical details for each and every

ophthalmic drug need to be known and will determine how the product should be used.

- **Nasal/bronchial administration.** This term describes drug administration across the nasal mucus epithelium and into the peripheral circulation. Many such pharmaceuticals are actually used for local treatment of the nasal mucosa (e.g. nasal decongestants), but the method is also used for systemic drug delivery. These pharmaceuticals are in the form of fine mists or vapours.

  The respiratory epithelia are an extension of the nasal mucosa and so the term also applies to pharmaceuticals administered for the bronchial system. These will be used for local therapeutic actions in the upper respiratory tract and take the form of sprays or finely dispersed powders that are administered via an inhaler or nebuliser.

- **Buccal/sublingual administration.** This term describes the administration of drugs across the buccal or lingual epithelia into the peripheral circulation. The pharmaceutical forms are usually lozenges, sprays or vapours.

- **Oral administration**, abbreviated po. Pharmaceuticals administered orally can enter the body via the buccal epithelia but predominantly are swallowed and then

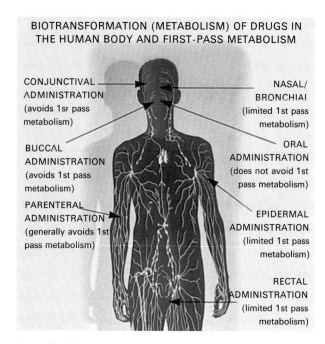

**Figure 1.13**
*Biotransformation (metabolism) of drugs in the human body with respect to first-pass metabolism. Metabolised drugs then leave the liver to reach the vital organs such as the heart.*

absorbed across the mucosa of the stomach and lower alimentary tract. Oral pharmaceuticals can take the form of solutions, elixirs (solutions with alcohol) and syrups as well as tablets (note ID/brand, pre-scoring (Pres-Tabs), colour coating, etc), capsules, gelcaps, caplets, sustained or slow-release tablets, etc.

- **Rectal administration**. This term is used both to imply use of pharmaceuticals for local therapy as well as for specific delivery of drugs, via the lower GI tract mucosal membranes into the peripheral circulation. Rectal pharmaceuticals usually take the form of suppositories but other insertion devices (including those containing gels), local creams, ointments, gels etc. are available.

- **Vaginal administration**. For local therapy of the vaginal mucus membranes only. Usually take the form of solutions (douches), creams, gels or various types of inserts.

- **Epidermal administration**. This term is used for administration of drugs across the dermis and absorption into the peripheral circulation. These pharmaceuticals can be used for local action or systemic drug delivery. The pharmaceuticals include creams, ointments, gels, powders (including wet or dry sprays) and special trans-dermal patch delivery systems including tapes, filters, pads and patches).

- **Parenteral administration**. This term means injection of a pharmaceutical which is a solution, so it might be simply designated as 'inj'. The delivery can be a single dose or continuous (e.g. intravenous drip). The injection site can be intravenous (iv), intramuscular (im), subcutaneous (sc), subconjunctival or intraocular. A retrobulbar injection is usually into the extraocular muscles or into the tissues surrounding these muscles but, in very special cases, injections are deliberately made into the optic nerve.

## The fate of drugs, from medicines, after administration

As noted above, there is a reason for the availability of the many different pharmaceuticals so that their routes of administration can be chosen to optimise drug delivery to its intended site of action. The various routes of administration are used to get maximum benefit from the natural circulation of the drug throughout the body (pharmacokinetics) after the pharmaceutical has been administered (Figure 1.13).

Some of the reasons are obvious in that for local therapy of some diseases or ailments it is logical to apply a local remedy. Skin ointment is applied to an abrasion, spray decongestants are used up the nose and eyedrops are used to relieve irritation of the conjunctiva.

However, for drug delivery to the inside of the body, the different routes are designed to optimise drug delivery to the target organ.[17,19] This optimisation is primarily related to the metabolism (biotransformation) of drugs in the human body. This metabolism of drugs primarily occurs in the liver.

Most medications are taken by the oral route and, as a result, are usually readily metabolised by the liver because the circulation around the GI tract leads straight to the liver via the hepatic portal system. As a result, a certain percentage of the absorbed drug (10–99%) is metabolised by the liver within minutes of being absorbed into the body. This process is called first-pass metabolism. When deciding how much drug is needed to manage any disease in the body, this first-pass metabolism has to be taken into account and that is why the pharmacokinetics are important.

This issue of biotransformation can be important and extend to pharmacy medicines. When two drugs are administered concurrently, one of them may impair this liver-based biotransformation of the other drug. As a result, the circulating levels of the non-metabolised form of one of the drugs may reach much higher levels than normally predicted from the pharmacokinetics. These elevated levels may constitute a form of overdose and could have substantial clinical consequences.

It is important to note that this first-pass metabolism largely can be avoided if the buccal, sublingual or rectal modes of administration are used, because the drug enters the peripheral circulation first and only then moves to the main circulation before then going to the liver. The same also applies to the conjunctival mode of delivery after systemic absorption of the drugs has occurred. This accounts for listed S/Ps on the use of sympathomimetic eyedrops (phenylephrine 10%) for example.

The selection of the buccal or sublingual routes is thus also a means to quickly achieve high concentrations of a designated drug in the circulation and at the target tissue since there is only limited loss of the drug before first-pass metabolism.

There are many reasons for the use of different pharmaceuticals. Some of these reasons are simply so that the actual mode of administration can be effected (see above). However, there are other reasons relating to optimisation of drug delivery for a particular mode of administration. For example, a normal tablet is designed to dissolve slowly in the stomach fluids and any drug administered orally has to be stable both to oral digestive enzymes and the acid pH of the stomach.

The same drug also has to be soluble in either gastric or duodenal fluids to be effectively absorbed into the body after oral administration. However, if the tablet is coated or is a slow/sustained-release tablet or caplet, then the dissolution will not occur until the pharmaceutical is about to leave the stomach. This ensures drug release is either slow and non-irritating to the stomach, or timed such that it occurs as the drug enters the lower alimentary tract.

In marked contrast, parenteral administration is generally used to administer a drug that cannot be given orally, either because it is unstable, e.g. insulin, or because it is necessary to get a drug into the tissues or circulation very fast.

Once pharmaceuticals are administered, the drugs in these pharmaceuticals are circulated round the body, and are then biotransformed and excreted.[17,19] Some form of metabolism or biotransformation is often necessary before a drug is excreted as its metabolite, especially via the urine. A drug metabolism usually initially results in a breakdown of the drug into an inactive metabolite, and this process is termed non-synthetic biotransformation.

As a second step, most initial drug metabolites are then metabolised further to change them into a chemical form that is optimum for excretion from the body. This second stage is usually termed synthetic biotransformation because the drug is derivatised; that is, molecular side chains are added to it. The non-synthetic biotransformation of a drug by the body does not always have to result in its inactivation. Some metabolites, as well as the initial drug, have biological activity. In fact, some pharmaceuticals are designed this way so that the drug has no biological activity until it is biotransformed by the body. These are called 'pro-drugs' and constitute an important aspect of modern pharmaceuticals.

Drugs may be used in this pro-drug form for a number of reasons – to increase bioavailability due to increased tissue penetration, or to allow site-specific delivery to cells or tissues in the body, but also to change the taste of a drug, to increase its stability.[20]

Last but not least, a drug will need to be excreted from the body. This process is called bioelimination.[17] Bioelimination occurs via several easily-identified routes:

- **Via the kidney.** The renal excretion route is generally the most important route for drug excretion. A substantial proportion (70%) of most drugs is eliminated from the body by this route. Obviously, if a patient has kidney malfunction, drug excretion is likely to be impaired and these patients are at risk of developing adverse effects from having too much residual drug in their bodies. This may be relevant even to the management of eye disease where, as the POM Livostin example given earlier showed, certain types of eyedrops should not be prescribed if a patient has renal impairment.

  It should also be realised that drugs which promote urinary output could increase bioelimination, thus necessitating more careful monitoring of patients' responses to the medication.

- **Via biliary and faecal routes.** Many drug metabolites are secreted into the intestinal tract via the bile fluids (through the spleen). After such internal excretion, these metabolites are eliminated in the faeces along with drugs administered orally that were never actually absorbed into the body. The metabolites are produced originally in the liver hepatocytes/ducts and then transferred to the bile system, rather than simply being transferred via the blood to the kidneys or to the rest of the body.

- **Via the saliva and sweat.** Small quantities of drugs and their metabolites can be excreted via these fluids. The quantities will depend on the magnitude of these physiological phenomena in a particular patient – if a drug promoted salivation or sweating, then more is likely to be eliminated via these routes.

- **Via the tears.** A little studied phenomenon but it can occur, and can be a cause of ocular irritation. Equally importantly, the phenomenon can sometimes be used to advantage in that a systemic drug can be 'delivered' to the conjunctiva via the tears.

- **Via breast milk.** Clinically, one should assume that any drug administered to a nursing mother can be transferred to her milk, and thus to her child. These drugs may be hazardous to the infant. The *BNF* or *MIMS* often contain statements as to whether the drugs in question should be taken by a nursing mother.

- **In the hair and skin.** Pigmented skin is more likely to accumulate drugs and their metabolites. Assessments of hair and skin samples can be used medically or in forensic sciences. A sustained accumulation of drugs in the skin can precipitate photosensitisation reactions.

There are some interesting anomalies to drug bioelimination. One of these relates to entero-hepatic shunting. This recognises that even though certain drugs, or their metabolites, are secreted in the bile after biotransformation in the liver, these metabolites can still be re-absorbed back into the body and enter the bloodstream again. These metabolites might then be excreted via the kidney or another route.

In chronic drug dosing, a unique phenomenon can occur, in some patients, even when normal excretion mechanisms appear to be operative. Some drugs (especially the heart drug digoxin, most synthetic corticosteroids and some antipsychotic drugs) readily undergo first-pass metabolism in the liver to produce active metabolites. These metabolites are secreted into the alimentary tract via the bile along with some of the original drug.

The secreted drug and metabolites are then re-absorbed into the body and are recycled back to the liver for another round of transformation and secretion. This cycling can go on for days or weeks and is called entero-hepatic shunting. It can result in unwanted and sustained medicinal effects, or adverse drug reactions that can persist for a long time after the medication has been discontinued.

## References

1 Opticians Act (1989) Chapter 44, and as now modified by Statutory Instrument 1999 No. 3267 (see Introduction).

2 Alexander D (1996) The shape of things to come. *Optician* **211**: 17.

3 Kerr C, Roberson G (1995) A matter of priority. *Optician* **209**: 18–19.

4 Department of Health (1999) *Review of Prescribing, Supply & Administration of Medicines. Final Report* (The Crown Report).

5 Doughty MJ (2000) *General Pharmacology for Primary Eye Care*, 2nd edn. Smawcastellane Information Services, Henry Bell St, Helensburgh G84 7HL, Scotland.

6 Optometrist's Formulary, 3rd edn. (1998) College of Optometrists, 42 Craven St., London WC2N 5NG.

7 The Medicines Act (1968) Chapter 67.

8 O'Conner Davies PH (1978) Medicines legislation and the ophthalmic optician. Reprint from *The Ophthalmic Optician* September 16 (4 pages).

9 *Chemist & Druggist Guide to OTC Medicines*. Miller Freeman UK Ltd., Sovereign Way, Tonbridge, Kent TN9 1RW, UK (tel. 01732-377487). Published yearly; individual copies are available.

10 *OTC Directory*. Proprietary Association of Great Britain (PAGB), Vernon House, Sicilian Ave., London WC1A 2QH. Published periodically; individual copies available from PAGB.

11 *MIMS (Monthly Index of Medical Specialities)*. Galleon Ltd, PO Box 219, Woking, Surrey GU21 1ZW, UK. Annual subscription rates available on request.

12 *BNF (British National Formulary)*. British Medical Association & Royal Pharmaceutical Society of Great Britain (RPSGB). Published bi-annually. Copies can be purchased from bookstores or from the RPSGB. Electronic version (eBNF) also available.

13 Doughty MJ (1999) Re-wetting, comfort, lubricant and moisturising solutions for the contact lens wearer. *Contact Lens Anterior Eye* **22**: 116–126.

14 Dale JR, Appelbe GE (1989) *Pharmacy Law and Ethics*, 4th edn. The Pharmaceutical Press, London.

15 ABPI Compendium of Data Sheets and Summaries of Product Characteristics. DataPharm Publications Ltd., 12 Whitehall, London SW1A 2DY, UK.

16 Shannon MT, Wilson BA, Stang CL (1995) *Govoni & Hayes Drugs and Nursing Implications*. Appleton & Lange, CT, USA.

17 Doughty MJ (1991) Basic Principles of pharmacology. In: *Clinical Ocular Pharmacology and Therapeutics* (Onofrey B, ed). JB Lippincott, Philadelphia Chapter 1, pp. 1–38.

18 Olejnik O (1993) Conventional systems in ophthalmic drug delivery. In: *Ophthalmic Drug Delivery Systems* (Mitra AK, ed). Marcel Dekker Inc., New York, USA, pp. 177–198.

19 Gibaldi M (1984) *Biopharmaceutics and Clinical Pharmacokinetics*. Lea & Febiger, Philadelphia, PA, USA.

20 Balant LP, Doelker E, Buri P (1990) Prodrugs for the improvement of drug absorption via different routes of administration. *Eur J Drug Metab Pharmacokin* **15**:143–153.

# 2

# Anatomy, neurophysiology and neuropharmacology of the eye

Anatomy of the eye
Innervation to intra- and extraocular structures
Mechanisms of drug interaction with nerves and nerve endplates
Drug delivery to the eye
Factors determining the efficacy of drug action on the eye

## Introduction

Evaluation of the actions of drugs on the eye requires consideration of the sites where drugs bind, and how the drugs get to these sites. The sites generally determine the selectivity of drug action because of the molecular mechanisms by which the drugs exert their particular effects. The principles of drug-receptor theory (pharmacodynamics) will be considered as they pertain to the clinical use of drugs, along with factors that affect the time-dependent response of the eye to both local and systemic drugs.

## Anatomy of the eye

Most attention is given usually to the cornea when considering drug delivery to the eye,[1–4] but there are five main aspects of ocular anatomy that need consideration:[5–7] the corneal epithelium; the structure of the conjunctival tissue; the puncta and nasolacrimal duct; the extraocular muscles and the orbital glands and their vascular supply; and the posterior vascular supply to the eye.

In addition there are the fine structural details of the intraocular tissue where the

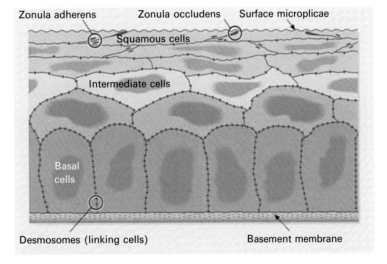

**Figure 2.1**
*Corneal epithelial ultrastructure showing the presence of zonula occludens as barriers to paracellular drug penetration.*

drugs act to produce physiological effects such as the iris muscles, the ciliary body muscles and zonule system, the ciliary epithelium and the uveo-scleral pathway (see Chapters 7 and 10).[5–7]

The ultrastructure of the corneal epithelium (Figure 2.1) represents a significant barrier to the penetration of drugs and other ingredients of pharmaceuticals into

the eye.[6] The barrier is probably the result of ultramicroscopic linkages both between the surface cells (the zonula occludens) and between the deeper-lying cells (desmosomes),[5] but can be readily altered *in vivo*[8] and *in vitro*[9] with loss of the most superficial cells. The normal barrier of the corneal epithelium can be demonstrated readily *in vivo*.

Sodium fluorescein solutions will form a coloured film across the healthy corneal surface and will take several minutes to permeate through the cornea.[7,8,10] The relative quantity of drugs that actually cross the cornea from ophthalmic pharmaceuticals is probably less than 1% of the total quantity in the pharmaceutical.[2,3,6,7] However, if the surface cells are compromised by repeated application of topical ocular anaesthetics, the surface will show punctate staining and the penetration of the fluorescein can be enhanced two- to fourfold.[8]

In cases of severe epitheliopathy, as in keratitis, it can be expected that no functional barrier exists and the drug(s) will penetrate up to 10 times faster.[3,7]

Topical ophthalmic pharmaceuticals are mainly water-soluble formulations of drugs (see Chapter 4) that eventually have to be miscible with the aqueous phase of the tear film before being able to penetrate into the eye.[3] These solubilised drugs can then slowly permeate between the corneal epithelial cells and ultimately enter the eye. Transcorneal drug transfer is aided, in part, by the fact that some drugs can also partition into the lipid phase of the corneal epithelial cells. In other words, they have lipophilic rather than hydrophilic characteristics.[3,6,7]

In dipivalyl epinephrine (dipivefrin, POM Propine), the valyl side-groups enhance corneal permeability. This pro-drug is then converted into the active drug, epinephrine, by esterase enzymes in the cornea. A similar principle is being developed for what are termed 'soft' drugs that are metabolised readily by the corneal or uveal tissue after tissue permeation.[2,6,7]

Notwithstanding, it is the properties of drugs in water that primarily determine corneal penetration, with the net ionic charge on the drug being the most important determinant. Drugs that possess a net positive or negative charge in the physiological pH range (pH 6.5 to 8.0) will permeate more slowly than uncharged drugs. Some drugs have no net charge despite having discrete charged chemical groups. This requires careful drug design which may take many years – for instance dorzolamide (POM Trusopt), developed from acetazolamide[6] (Chapter 10).

Another important determinant of the corneal penetration is the time the pharmaceutical is in contact with the corneal surface. This contact time can be enhanced

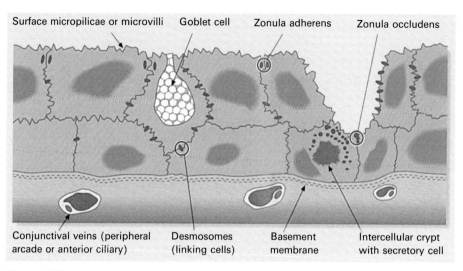

**Figure 2.2**
*The conjunctival tissue showing the presence of zonula adherens as barriers to parcellular drug penetration.*

two or three times by the use of pharmaceuticals containing 'viscolisers' (see Chapter 4).[3,6,10]

Overall, the corneal epithelial barrier is more important in eyes mildly compromised by chronic allergic conjunctivitis (or similar); the repeated application of eye drops containing even low concentrations of drugs could result in unexpectedly high intraocular levels of drugs, precipitating unwanted side-effects.[10]

Conjunctiva tissue structure (Figure 2.2) is recognised nowadays as an important site of drug delivery,[3,6,7,11] with its permeability to drugs being some twofold higher than the cornea.[11] The superficial epithelial cell arrays across the bulbar and palpebral conjunctiva probably have a similar barrier structure to the corneal epithelium,[5–7] and it appears likely that the permeation of drugs into the conjunctival tissue will be determined by similar characteristics to those for corneal penetration.[6,7,11] However, the conjunctival surfaces also contain numerous secretory cells and glands, which could have a substantial impact on net drug absorption.[12]

The transconjunctival drug permeation is important for the action of topical ocular vasoconstrictor drugs (for instance naphazoline in P Murine) or topical ocular corticosteroids for conjunctival inflammation (such as clobetasone in POM Cloburate) at the superficial and deeper conjunctival vasculature (see Chapter 6). The conjunctival

cell barrier to drug penetration can be overcome easily by injecting drug solution into the conjunctival tissue.[7,11] Such subconjunctival injection is used in the specialist management of intraconjunctival inclusions such as chalazia with corticosteroids, or hyperacute infections with antibiotics.

The transconjunctival absorption of drugs from ophthalmic pharmaceuticals is also a selective site for systemic absorption of drugs such as cyclopentolate.[6,11] This route to the anterior ciliary veins and the periocular vasculature and the intraorbital venous return is important, since such absorption will not be 'blocked' by eyelid closure or punctal occlusion.

Nasolacrimal drainage (Figure 2.3A) is the ultimate and inescapable fate of ophthalmic pharmaceuticals, unless there is substantial blockage of the puncta and nasolacrimal duct. This site's impact on ocular pharmacokinetics is often misrepresented. Under normal circumstances, an ophthalmic pharmaceutical solution will drain rapidly through the open puncta,[3,7,11] and through the nasolacrimal duct for absorption through the epithelial mucosa lining the duct into the nasal and then facial vasculature, with the highest absorption probably for uncharged drugs and similar to that of the conjunctiva.[11]

The rapid drainage can be visualised by gamma scintography, in which eye drops are labelled with the non-toxic radiochemical [99]Tc technetium to illustrate the

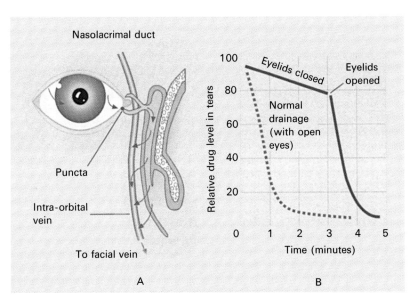

**Figure 2.3**
*Nasolacrimal drainage to the intraocular vascular supply (A) and schematic representation of the kinetics of nasolacrimal drainage of ophthalmic pharmaceuticals with and without simple eyelid closure (B).*

effects of viscolisers on slowing down the rate of drainage.[3,11] Since punctal patency requires open eyelids, it should not be surprising that gently closing the eyelids should slow down the rate of drainage, and that this will resume promptly as soon as the eyelids are re-opened (Figure 2.3B).[13]

Eyelid closure (for at least one minute) can improve greatly the efficacy of ophthalmic products containing drugs such as timolol[14] (e.g. POM Timoptol), and should be used regularly to promote corneal absorption of all therapeutic eye drops.

The extraocular muscles, orbital glands and their vascular supply (Figure 2.4) are affected by systemic medications (Chapter 7). These muscles have a unique combination of striated and smooth muscle types, and a substantial blood supply also linked to the main lacrimal glands.[5,15] A peripheral arterial arcade from the facial artery is located above the tarsal plate and palpebral muscles, and also supplies the underlying conjunctiva. There is also an indirect supply from the lacrimal branch of the ophthalmic artery to the orbital glands, which further branches to the lateral palpebral arteries deeper within the eyelid and conjunctiva.

Deeper lying branches of anterior ciliary artery supply both the rectus muscles and ultimately the bulbar conjunctiva. The eyelid and orbital vasculature form another type of barrier between drugs and their absorption. Fenestrated or non-fenestrated capillaries can be expected to be relatively impermeable to drugs but slow transendothelial permeation can occur. The principles of such permeation can be expected to follow those of the blood–brain barrier[16] and the posterior blood–eye barrier (see below). Drug penetration is again influenced by charge and lipophilic properties.

The posterior vascular arcade (Figure 2.5) can also effectively deliver drugs to the eye. Transcorneal and some transconjunctival (scleral) penetration of drugs from topical ophthalmic pharmaceuticals might be considered the most substantial route of drug delivery to the eye. However, the systemic administration of medicines will result in delivery of many drugs to the eye.[7]

The choroidal space and the anterior uvea are supplied by branches of the short posterior ciliary arteries (principally to the choroid) and of the long posterior ciliary arteries (principally to the anterior uvea, and ultimately to the conjunctival–scleral boundary). Some smaller branches of the anterior ciliary arteries also supply the anterior choroid. The combined anterior blood supply is a route by which drugs from systemic medications can enter the eye and affect secretory functions to alter IOP (Chapter 10).

The most anterior arterial branches to bulbar (and palpebral) conjunctiva deliver oral drugs (such as histamine $H_1$ drugs)[17] to this tissue. The principal barrier to delivery of systemic drugs is presumably the vascular endothelia, which can be

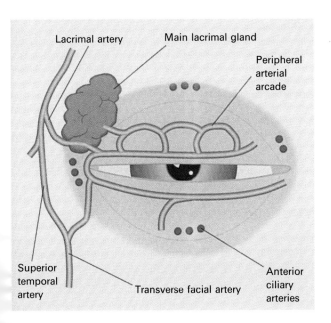

**Figure 2.4**
*The extraocular muscles, extraorbital lacrimal glands and their vascular supply for transfer of drugs from the systemic circulation.*

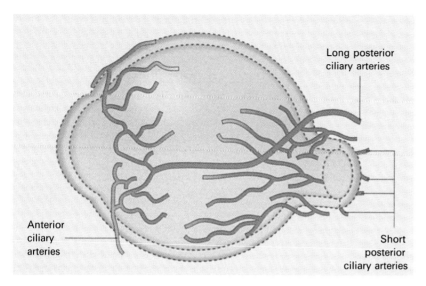

**Figure 2.5**
*The posterior arterial supply to the eye permitting delivery of drugs from the systemic circulation to the choroid and anterior uvea.*

compromised readily with resultant emigration of inflammatory cells and other blood constituents into the eye tissue.[7,10] This blood-aqueous barrier can be modulated by topical ocular corticosteroids and non-steroidal anti-inflammatory drugs (NSAIDs).[7,10]

This vascular permeability can also be decreased directly and indirectly by other vasoactive drugs such as cholinergic blockers, for instance homatropine eye drops. The selective use of these drugs constitutes an important part of management of ocular inflammation and the postoperative patient (see Chapter 6). Lastly, and more recently recognised, is the overall permeability of the uveal tissue to fluid and drugs (the uveoscleral route) that is important in the efficacy of antiglaucoma drugs, such as the prostaglandin $F_2$ analogue, latanoprost (POM Xalatan).[18]

## Innervation to intra- and extraocular structures

Both the external and internal eye are richly innervated.[1,5,15] Traditionally, attention has been given primarily to the parasympathetic (cholinergic) and sympathetic (adrenergic) nerves that are found in abundance in the pupil, anterior vasculature and ciliary body.

However, just as a range of other neurotransmitters is found in the CNS (see Chapter 3), it should also be recognised that there is autonomic innervation to main lacrimal glands, and that the anterior eye innervation also includes histaminergic, serotoninergic and peptidergic (substance P) receptors involved in various types of nocioception and pain.[19] There is also evidence that special peptidergic nerves, including VIP (vasoactive intestinal peptide) and CGRP (calcitonin gene-related peptide), regulate conjunctival goblet cells and meibomian glands.

## Mechanisms of drug interaction with nerves, nerve endplates and other receptors

The overall mechanism of action (the pharmacodynamics) of a drug generally distinguishes a medication containing drugs from a chemical that is causing a toxic reaction. Pharmacodynamics describe the molecular action of a drug and the overall principles for defining them are well established as the basis of the clinical action of a drug.

Practitioner-oriented pharmaceutical directories (see Chapter 1) often contain a section called the 'pharmacology of a drug'. This pharmacological profile will include details of the mode of administration (the pharmaceutics), the time base and magnitude of drug action after administration (the pharmacokinetics) and the

mechanism of action of the drug (the pharmacodynamics) by which it is usually classified – for instance as an antihistamine, or more specifically, a histamine $H_1$ blocking drug or antagonist.

When a pharmaceutical is administered to the surface of the eye, injected or presented by other systemic routes, the drug in the pharmaceutical will end up at discrete locations that are the sites of action. In cellular and molecular terms, these sites of action can be referred to generally as 'receptors', which are binding sites for drugs. Receptors can be proteins that are present on cells in a tissue (for instance for histamine $H_1$ blocking drugs such as antazoline in P Otrivine–Antistin) or within cells (for antibacterial drugs on ribosomes such as chloramphenicol in POM Chloromycetin).

Drug binding can also be to the active site of enzymes present in the fluids of the body, in membranes of cells or inside cells (to carbonic anhydrase for dorzolamide in POM Trusopt, for example). Lastly, the drug binding can be to sites that are less well defined but represent an important therapeutic target. Examples here would include cell membranes which show a strong association with drugs to block electrophysiological activity (for topical ocular anaesthetics such as amethocaine) or increase the overall permeability of a membrane (polymyxin B in POM PolyFax for bacterial membranes).

Drug binding to proteinaceous receptors is assessed easily either by drug-binding studies, or from dose-dependent modulation of receptor-related function (Figure 2.6). The drug action may either be to mimic the action of the neurotransmitter (phenylephrine binding to alpha-adrenergic receptors, for instance), or to block the action of the neurotransmitter or other biological modulator (the antazoline in P Otrivine–Antistin is an example of a histamine $H_1$ blocking drug).

For drug binding to enzymes, inhibition or stimulation of the enzyme activity can be measured *in vitro*, or the dose-dependent modulation of a function such as IOP (Figure 2.7). Dose-dependent drug interaction with membranes can be measured from electrophysiological studies, or from modulation of functions such as corneal sensitivity.

There has long been an application of this receptor theory to the autonomic nervous system and the eye,[1,4] in that it has been recognised that there are proteinaceous

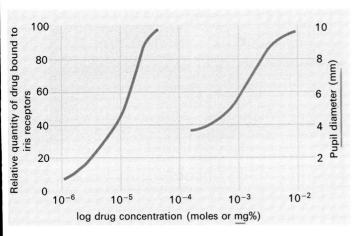

**Figure 2.6**
*Idealised presentation of the binding of an adrenergic drug to adrenergic alpha₁ receptors of the iris (green) and dose-dependence of modulation of pupil diameter (red).*

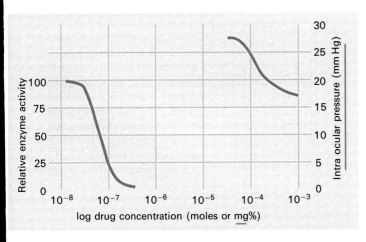

**Figure 2.7**
*Idealised presentation of the inhibition of carbonic anhydrase activity of ciliary epithelial tissues by a carbonic anhydrase inhibitor (green) and dose-dependence of reduction of IOP (red).*

drug, whether 10%, 50% or 100%. The concentration range at which many of the 'receptors' have bound the drug has great medicinal relevance and is usually equated with the 50% 'receptor' binding. From a molecular perspective, this 50% drug binding is called the Kd and is a quantitative measure of the affinity of the drug for the receptor.[4] In clinical terms, the drug quantity that generally needs to be administered is that which essentially produces a 50% binding and thus a 50% activity effect. This effective dose is thus known as the ED$_{50}$ (*ee-dee-fifty*).

Since there will usually be a defined range of concentrations over which a drug receptor or target site will operate under the influence of a drug, this concentration range determines the drug dose given to a patient. The drug can either bind directly to a receptor and produce an effect or can bind to a site on the receptor such that it either displaces another drug or allows another drug to bind more readily. The drug concentration that produces a 50% increase in binding of a second drug or that produces a 50% decrease in the binding of a second drug can be determined; the latter 50% effect is called an inhibitory 50% or I$_{50}$ (*eye-fifty*).

If the drug interacts with a membrane, the concentration–effect relationships are not so well defined. However, a concentration which produces a minimum or threshold effect can be measured from electrophysiological measurements on nerves and a concentration can be determined where there is a saturating effect on the nerve membranes. In the first case, just detectable anaesthesia would be produced and in the second case a total loss of sensation (or nerve block) would result. If the membrane were on a bacterium, a minimal concentration just producing an effect on the viability of the microorganisms over 24 hours can be determined as the minimum inhibitory concentration (MIC) or that concentration killing 90% of the organisms determined (LD$_{90}$).[4]

Since the drug is usually able to 'recognise' its receptor over only a certain concentration range, the drug has a unique 'affinity' for its receptor. If the concentration of the drug at which this recognition occurs is low, the drug is a potent one, and *vice versa*. As an example, miotic drugs have different affinities for their cholinergic receptors, especially when compared with the natural neurotransmitter acetylcholine

receptors for drugs such as phenylephrine and pilocarpine on the iris muscles, that there are enzymes mediating the biotransformation of adrenaline and acetylcholine in the iris tissue, and also enzymes for the biotransformation of phenylephrine (e.g. monoamine oxidase) and pilocarpine (pilocarpine esterase).[7] While the binding sites for membrane-active drugs remain poorly characterised,[4,10] a set of general principles can be applied.

The determination of drug binding or interaction with its sites of action is the basis of pharmacodynamics. Any drug action can be defined by its concentration-dependent effects when mixed with a 'receptor', or presented to the receptor in the living body. The dose–response plots (Figures 2.6 and 2.7) have been presented deliberately in logarithmic form for the dose (Figure 2.8). With the quantity of drug presented as a log function, it can be seen that there is a concentration when the drug shows just a small ability to bind to the 'receptor' (and produce a threshold activation or inhibition), a concentration where many of the 'receptors' will bind the drug easily and a concentration at which all of the drug 'receptors' have bound the drug (a plateau or saturation effect).

These concentrations can be measured in what are called drug-binding studies, which allow one to define the percentage of the receptors that have interacted with the

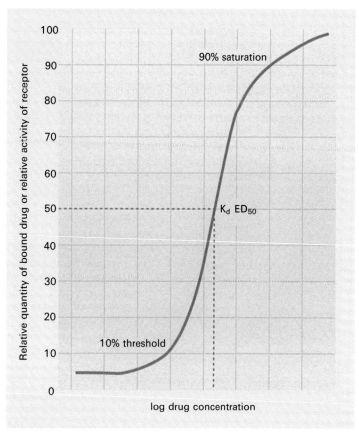

**Figure 2.8**
*Idealised presentation of drug interaction with a receptor.*

potency of a drug simply because many factors determine its action beyond it being able to bind to a receptor. The shift in the curves in Figures 2.6 and 2.7, when comparing the drug action at the receptor and the physiological effects, reflect the large differences between the administered dose and the quantity of drug reaching the receptors. Thus, in clinical terms, the term efficacy is used to describe the magnitude of drug effects.

A potent drug will generally show a high or substantial efficacy and *vice versa*, but this does not mean that a less potent drug cannot display high efficacy if administered at high enough doses. For example, the clinical efficacy of antiglaucoma pharmaceuticals, even if with different receptor mechanisms, could still be compared with timolol 0.5% *bds* as having higher (pilocarpine 2%, *qds*) or lower (adrenaline 1%, *tds*) efficacy (Figure 2.10).

Drugs generally either 'activate' or 'inhibit' receptor site(s). The drug interaction with a receptor can thus generally produce a positive or agonist effect (with the activity mediated via that receptor site being augmented), or the drug interaction can produce a negative or antagonist effect (with the activity mediated via that receptor being attenuated).

Agonist drugs can also be called mimetics or stimulants, and antagonist drugs can be referred to as lytics or blocking drugs. In the laboratory and clinical practice, agonists and antagonists can be used in various ways. For example, acetylcholine

(Figure 2.9). If two drugs that can act on the same receptor are presented simultaneously to the receptor, the more potent (or high affinity) drug will generally displace that which is less potent (or weak affinity). This applies regardless of whether the drugs 'activate' or 'inhibit' the receptor.

Clinically, one rarely refers to the

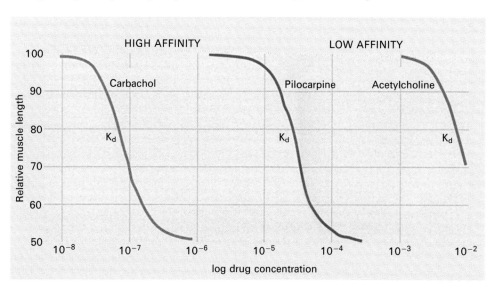

**Figure 2.9**
*Comparisons of drug potency from the binding and resultant contraction of the iris sphincter muscle* in vitro.

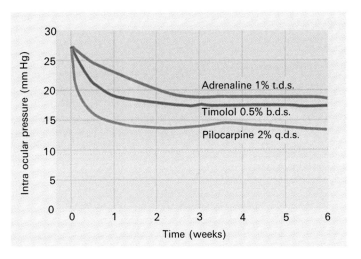

**Figure 2.10**
*Comparisons of pharmaceutical efficacy from the time-dependent lowering of IOP. The different pharmaceuticals (drugs) produce different hypotensive effects (different efficacy) even at similar concentrations.*

applied to an iris muscle preparation will cause it to contract. If echothiophate is also present, the concentration of acetylcholine needed to contract the muscle will be much less because the acetylcholine breakdown is inhibited by the echothiophate acting as an indirect agonist.[1,4]

Alternatively, an agonist drug effect can be counteracted by an antagonist (and *vice versa*) so that phenylephrine 2.5% can dilate the pupil via a direct action on alpha$_1$ adrenergic receptors, while thymoxamine can close the pupil via a direct blocking action on the same receptors.[20]

Such agonist–antagonist interaction is not always demonstrable, not because it does not occur but because the overall physiological processes are not well understood. For example, high concentrations of the beta-adrenergic agonists adrenaline or isoproterenol can be expected to displace beta-adrenergic blocking drugs such as timolol from their ciliary receptors, yet all three drugs will lower IOP.

Drug actions at sites in the eye are the result of their interaction with receptors over a discrete concentration range. Some drugs have similarities in molecular structure and will bind to a particular receptor over different discrete concentration ranges, depending on their affinity for that receptor (see Figures 2.6, 2.7 and 2.9). Drugs that have a different molecular structure will not bind, but drugs with a similar molecular structure may bind. Drug action can thus be selective, based both on concentration and molecular structure.

For the example of the antiglaucoma drugs, timolol will bind and block the aqueous secretion-related activity at both beta$_1$- and beta$_2$-adrenergic receptors in the ciliary epithelium and the uveal vasculature, while betaxolol should more selectively block only beta$_1$-receptors. In contrast, while the true mechanisms of IOP reduction remain a relative mystery, adrenaline should bind to all adrenergic receptors as a non-selective agonist, the drug apraclonidine should activate only alpha$_2$-receptors and reduce IOP. Conversely, phenylephrine as an alpha$_1$-adrenergic receptor agonist, should neither bind to beta-adrenergic receptors nor affect IOP significantly.

## Drug delivery to the eye

The action of any drug on ocular receptors depends on whether the drug was effectively delivered to those receptors. Equally importantly from a clinical perspective, it is important that the drug is then inactivated and removed from the eye. This delivery and removal determine the time base and magnitude of drug action, i.e. its pharmacokinetics.

After use of most ocular pharmaceuticals, various physiological functions of the eye are temporarily changed as a result of the drug binding. In addition, since the drug–receptor interaction is very much determined by the concentration of the drug in the vicinity of the receptors, there are distinct time-dependent alterations in receptor function concomitant with changes in drug concentrations in the vicinity of the receptor(s). That these concentrations will change is determined by the rates of drug movement (delivery) to the sites where the receptors are present, and by the rates of drug movement away from the receptors (see Chapter 1).

Such pharmacokinetics are perhaps best appreciated by considering systemic drug delivery to the eye (Figure 2.11A).

After systemic absorption of a drug from a medication (an oral antihistamine such as chlorpheniramine as in P Piriton, for example), the normal blood flow initially carries the drug into the eye and to conjunctival receptor sites. However, just as fast as the blood flow delivers the drug, it is also removing the drug to other parts of the body (where there are also receptors to bind the drug). In addition, some of the drug will be delivered simultaneously by the blood supply to the liver (for biotransformation) and to the kidney (for excretion from the body). As the minutes pass, the relative amount of the drug being delivered to the conjunctiva will get less and less as the drug is biotransformed and eliminated.

The whole process of drug delivery, absorption and wash-out is described by the pharmacokinetics and can be determined by making measurements of drug levels in different parts of the body after a pharmaceutical is administered. Systemically administered chlorpheniramine will pass by the conjunctiva at clinically relevant levels (to effect H$_1$ receptor blockade after conjunctival absorption) for 2–4 hours.[17]

It will also enter the extraocular muscles and lacrimal system, and the inside of the eye to have other effects on coordinated eye movement, lacrimation and pupil activity (see Chapters 5, 7 and 10). Any drug that actually enters the eye will follow a posterior-to-anterior route, eventually to leave the eye primarily by the trabecular route.[3,7]

A similar kinetic description can be applied to topical pharmaceuticals for another histamine H$_1$ receptor blocking drug such as antazoline (Figure 2.11B). After transconjunctival (or transcorneal) absorption, the drug will enter the anterior ocular tissue and aqueous humour and

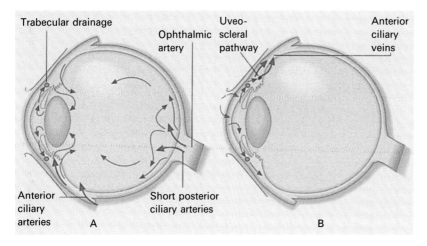

**Figure 2.11**
*Schematic representation of the overall process of drug delivery to and elimination from the inside of the eye after systemic administration (A) and after topical administration (B).*

have anterior effects, but should not move more posteriorly in the phakic eye – the crystalline lens and vitreous face, coupled with the normal direction of aqueous flow, serve as an effective 'barrier'.

In the post-surgical aphakic eye, this barrier is removed and aqueous flow is often diminished such that drugs can diffuse more posteriorly and have effects on the retinal nerve layers and superficial retinal vasculature,[7] for instance topical adrenaline-induced maculopathy.[21]

## Factors determining the efficacy of drug action on the eye

A number of general factors can affect drug pharmacokinetics. These are well known for systemically administered pharmaceuticals but also apply to the local delivery of drugs to the eye. The efficacy of drugs following systemic drug delivery is known to be determined by several secondary factors (see Table 2.1).

Effective drug absorption after oral administration requires a healthy alimentary tract with the volume of distribution (Chapter 1) being determined by good circulation. Biotransformation of many drugs requires a healthy liver, while bioelimination requires a normally functioning alimentary tract and kidney.

Other forms of drug–drug interactions (INT) can precipitate adverse drug reactions (ADRs) and prompt contraindications

---

**Table 2.1  Major factors affecting the efficacy of orally administered drugs**

The health of the alimentary tract
The health of the circulation
Rates of liver-based biotransformation
Rates of kidney-based bioelimination
Drug–drug interactions
Other substances (food, alcohol, illicit drugs)
Patient age and body mass
Pharmacogenetic factors
Chronopharmacological factors

---

(C/I) or specific precautions (S/P) for use of the drug. Possible interaction with the oral antihypertension drug, clonidine (POM Catapres), is listed for xylometazoline–antazoline eyedrops, but it should also be considered that hypertensive patients may exhibit erratic pharmacokinetics for oral or topical antihistamines. Other drugs may promote or reduce bioelimination of another drug, for instance diuretics such as hydrochlorothiazide (POM Hydrosaluric) promote urinary output and thus bioelimination of many drugs.

The presence of other substances from certain types of food, alcohol and illicit drugs can impair bioavailability and lead to unpredictable rates of biotransformation and bioelimination. As an example, the efficacy of absorption of oral tetracycline antibiotics (used for management of inclu-

sion conjunctivitis) can be reduced by milk and certain vegetables.

The age of patients is important, especially the very young versus the very old. From a systemic perspective, differences in the volume of distribution (very young patients) or the rates of biotransformation (the elderly) can result in different drug pharmacokinetics. The age effects can be indirect. For xylometazoline–antazoline eyedrops, the recommended dose is lower for elderly patients because of a higher risk of there being enhanced corneal penetration, and thus adverse reactions such as mydriasis.

Pharmacogenetics reflects the fact that some individuals metabolise drugs faster or slower than other individuals, or develop ADRs due to unique drug metabolism.[20] Such considerations probably underlie the reason why a small number of individuals develop severe aplastic anaemia to systemic or topical chloramphenicol,[10] and develop severe optic nerve damage from systemic antituberculosis drugs such as isoniazid.[22]

Chronopharmacology is the least-recognised aspect of drug delivery, but some drugs can have markedly different effects when administered at different times of the day. Topical ocular beta-blockers, for instance, have their greatest effect during the day.[23]

## References

1  Hopkins GA, Pearson RM (eds) (1998) General pharmacological principles. In: *O'Connor Davies's Ophthalmic Drugs: Diagnostic and Therapeutic Uses*, 5th edn. Butterworth-Heinemann, Oxford, UK.

2  Sasaki H, Yamamura K, Nishida K *et al.* (1996) Delivery of drugs to the eye by topical application. *Progr Retinal Eye Res* **15**: 583–620.

3  Olejnik O (1993) Conventional systems in ophthalmic drug delivery. In: *Ophthalmic Drug Delivery Systems* (Mitra AK, ed). Marcel Dekker Inc., New York, USA, pp. 177–198.

4  Doughty MJ (1991) Basic principles of pharmacology. In: *Clinical Ocular Pharmacology and Therapeutics* (Onofrey B, ed). JB Lippincott, Philadelphia, USA Chapter 1, pp. 1–38.

5  Jacobiec FA (1982) *Ocular Anatomy, Embryology and Teratology*. Harper & Row, Philadelphia, PA, USA.

6 Jarvinen K, Jarvinel T, Urtti A (1995) Ocular absorption following topical delivery. *Adv Drug Delivery Rev* **16**: 3–19.

7 Maurice DM, Mishima S (1984) Ocular pharmacokinetics. In: *Handbook Experimental Pharmacology* (Sears ML, ed). Springer-Verlag, Berlin, Germany, pp. 19–116.

8 Ramselaar JAM, Boot JP, Van Haeringen NJ *et al.* (1988) Corneal epithelial permeability after instillation of ophthalmic solutions containing local anaesthetics and preservatives. *Curr Eye Res* **7**: 947–950.

9 Doughty MJ (1995) Evaluation of the effects of saline versus bicarbonate-containing mixed-salts solutions on rabbit corneal epithelium in vitro. *Ophthal Physiol Opt* **15**: 585–599.

10 Doughty MJ (1996) Diagnostic and therapeutic pharmaceutical agents for use in contact lens practice. In: *Clinical Contact Lens Practice* (Bennett ED, Weissman BA, eds). JB Lippincott, Philadelphia, USA Chapter 9, pp. 1–38.

11 Urtti A, Salminen L (1993) Minimizing systemic absorption of topically administered ophthalmic drugs. *Surv Ophthalmol* **37**: 435–456.

12 Doughty MJ (1997) Scanning electron microscopy study of the tarsal and orbital conjunctival surfaces compared to peripheral corneal epithelium in pigmented rabbits. *Doc Ophthalmol* **93**: 345–371.

13 White WL, Glover AT, Buckner AB (1991) Effects of blinking on tear elimination as evaluated by dacryoscintography. *Ophthalmology* **98**: 367–369.

14 Ellis PP, Wu P-Y, Pfoff DS *et al.* (1992) Effect of nasolacrimal occlusion on timolol concentrations in the aqueous humor of the human eye. *J Pharm Sci* **81**: 219–220.

15 Dartt DA (1992) Physiology of tear production. In: *The Dry Eye* (Lemp MA, Marquardt R, eds). Springer-Verlag, Berlin, pp. 65–99.

16 Vinores SA (1995) Assessment of blood-retinal barrier integrity. *Histol Histopathol* **10**: 141–154.

17 Ciprandi G, Buscaglia S, Cerquetti PM *et al.* (1992) Drug treatment of allergic conjunctivitis. A review of the evidence. *Drugs* **43**: 154–176.

18 Toris CB, Camras CB, Yablonski ME (1993) Effect of PhXA41, a new prostaglandin $F_{2\alpha}$ analogue, on aqueous humor dynamics in human eyes. *Ophthalmology* **100**: 1297–1304.

19 Doughty MJ (1998) The pathological response of the anterior eye. *Optometry Today* Feb 13, pp. 28–32.

20 Doughty MJ, Lyle WM (1992) A review of the clinical pharmacokinetics of pilocarpine, moxisylyte (thymoxamine) and dapiprazole in the reversal of diagnostic pupillary dilation. *Optom Vis Sci* **69**: 358–368.

21 Classe JG (1980) Epinephrine maculopathy. *J Am Optom Assoc* **51**: 1091–1093.

22 Doughty MJ, Lyle WM (1992) Ocular pharmacogenetics. In: *Genetics for Primary Eye Care Practitioners* (Fatt HV, Griffin JR, Lyle WM, eds). Butterworth-Heinemann, Toronto, Canada, pp. 179–193.

23 Topper JE, Brubaker RF (1985) Effects of timolol, epinephrine, and acetazolamide on aqueous flow during sleep. *Invest Ophthalmol Vis Sci* **26**: 1315–1319.

# 3
# Neuropharmacology of the central and autonomic nervous system

The CNS vs the peripheral nervous system
Adrenaline-mediated neurotransmission
Acetylcholine-mediated neurotransmission
Serotonin-mediated neurotransmission
Dopamine-mediated neurotransmission
GABA-mediated neurotransmission
Histamine-mediated neurotransmission
Summary of medications for the CNS and their use
General impact of CNS drugs on the eye and vision

## Introduction

It is well known that the drugs contained in eyedrops used for diagnostic purposes produce specific effects on neurotransmitter receptors in the eye, i.e. through interaction with the peripheral or autonomic nervous system.[1,2] In exceptional circumstances, the unwanted systemic absorption of these drugs (see Chapter 2) can result in sufficient drug levels in the central nervous system (CNS) to produce adverse drug reactions (ADRs), for instance for cyclopentolate.[3]

Equally importantly, a large number of systemic medications contain drugs that are intended to produce CNS-based effects but can have a substantial range of effects on the eye, vision and oculomotor functions. While these interactions (INT) tend to be labelled as ADRs, it should be recognised that many of these effects are merely the expected consequences of specific CNS pathway activation (or blockade).

Knowledge of CNS-active medications is very important (Table 3.1). CNS-based

> ### Table 3.1   When details of medications active within the CNS need to be available
>
> - Prior to the use of certain therapeutic drugs for IOP (adrenaline, beta-blockers, guanethidine, apraclonidine, brimonidine)
> - Prior to the use of certain therapeutic drugs for ocular inflammation (xylometazoline, antazoline, levocabastine, atropine, homatropine, oral antihistamines)
> - Prior to the use of neuroactive diagnostic ophthalmic drugs (mydriatics and cycloplegics)
> - As part of a differential diagnosis of symptomatic patients
> - For all patients who are subjected to tests that require stereopsis, or at least reasonable binocular single vision (including visual fields)
> - As part of the assessment of patients with any form of binocular coordination problems

systemic medications need to be considered as part of a differential diagnosis of symptomatic patients and to be considered very carefully in the assessment of patients with any form of binocular coordination problems (including when such patients are subjected to tests that require stereopsis, or at least reasonable binocular single vision).

Equally importantly, the history of such drug use should be known about before the use of neuroactive diagnostic ophthalmic drugs (mydriatics and cycloplegics) and prior to the use of neuroactive drugs for intraocular pressure (IOP) (adrenaline, beta-blockers, guanethidine, apraclonidine, brimonidine) or ocular inflammation (xylometazoline, antazoline, levocabastine, atropine, homatropine, oral antihistamines). It is the intent of this chapter to detail the CNS sites of action of these drugs, their neurotransmitters and why they can have substantial impact on the eye.

The mechanisms by which systemic drugs interact with the eye and CNS are important. These drugs can bind to receptors, or change the levels of the neurotransmitters that are available to interact naturally with their receptors. The former group of drugs is more likely to produce transient but potentially substantial effects on the eye and could even constitute ocular emergencies. The latter group of indirect-acting drugs is more likely to produce recurrent, longer-term but perhaps more subtle effects on the eye and vision. Furthermore, some of these drugs have multiple sites of action and are thus more likely to precipitate ADRs.

## Overview of the CNS vs the peripheral nervous system

For each organ or tissue, it is accepted that there are subtle differences in the known balances between the effects of adrenergic vs cholinergic drug effects simply because each site has its own particular balance of sympathetic and parasympathetic innervation. Part of this overall balance is also determined by the CNS by excitatory or inhibitory controls, and involves other neurotransmitters such as serotonin, dopamine, GABA and histamine.

Inter-relationships between the pathways are important because the different brain centres that are linked to peripheral organs (including the eye) are generally separately amenable to drug action to produce both central and peripheral actions. Subtle-to-substantial end-organ effects, including at the eye, can thus be expected.

For consideration of CNS-related drug action, it is important that the potential complexity of the synaptic transmission mechanisms be realised. Such a complexity is summarised in Figure 3.1. For such nerve–nerve, nerve–muscle or nerve–gland transmission, there are two essential components; the pre- and post-synaptic cells.

The process of junctional transmission is initiated by the arrival of an action potential (or sequence of action potentials) at the pre-junctional cells. The resultant changes in electrical potential difference that occur within the pre-synaptic axon cell then promote the release of an excitatory or an

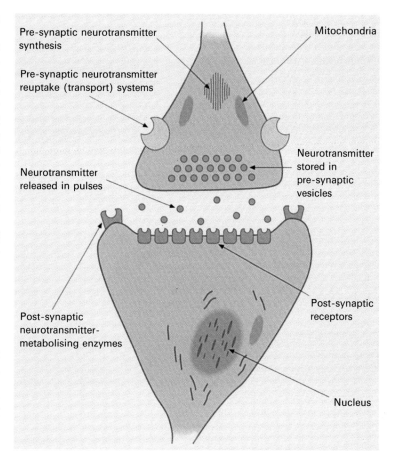

**Figure 3.1**
*Components of a nerve–nerve synaptic junction.*

inhibitory neurotransmitter chemical from vesicles in the terminal into the synapse (the synaptic cleft). While details for all the CNS systems are not available, it is likely that all include distinct steps for the synthesis and storage of the neurotransmitters and a specific mechanism for release of the neurotransmitters.

The same pre-synaptic cell is likely to store and release only a single neurotransmitter substance of the types considered in this module. In the simplest case, these neurotransmitters are released in pulses, will then diffuse across the synaptic cleft, following which they can briefly interact with post-synaptic receptors. Various types of biotransformation processes then inactivate them.

These biotransformation processes can occur on the post-synaptic side (e.g. acetylcholinesterase and catecholamine-O-methyl transferase), or within the pre-synaptic terminals, especially in the mitochondria (e.g. for catecholamines).

However, with many currently used drugs, the situation is complicated by specific neurotransmitter-selective pre-synaptic reuptake mechanisms (that in themselves are regulated by the actual levels of neurotransmitter originally released).

There are also specific receptor-mediated pathways that block further transmitter release; these are (bio)feedback mechanisms which can involve different 'autoreceptor' receptor (sub)types to those involved in the actual neurotransmission events. Lastly, the biotransformation of CNS-active drugs can produce active metabolites that have recurring secondary actions to sustain or further modulate the neurotransmission.

At appropriately determined dosage ranges, direct-acting drugs will produce their clinically-relevant effects until they dissociate from the receptors and are then reabsorbed, biotransformed and eliminated. Indirect-acting neuroactive drugs are just as widely used, if not more widely used, in the population at large and change the way in which the neurotransmitters are released, reabsorbed or biotransformed. While the clinical end-result of the use of indirect-acting drugs is often similar to that for direct-acting drugs, the time base of drug action can be quite different and provides the clinician with an important option for medication strategy.

## Noradrenaline-mediated neurotransmission

Sympathetic effects are produced by noradrenaline (norepinephrine) and adrenaline (epinephrine), both classified as catecholamines. The principal noradrenaline pathways in the CNS ascend from the brainstem to the hypothalamus and forebrain. Noradrenaline is actually synthesised in nerve terminals from another catecholamine called dopamine, and in some terminals the noradrenaline will then be used for the synthesis of adrenaline, giving different catecholamine synapses.

The neurotransmitter released at nerve endings in muscles or glands is usually noradrenaline, while adrenaline is produced by the adrenal glands and circulates in our blood and in parts of the CNS (and so determines blood flow to the CNS and body).

Noradrenaline, adrenaline or direct-acting adrenergic drugs generally bind to adrenergic receptors to augment the actual function of the receptor. However, this augmentation can have opposite physiological consequences depending on whether the receptor is an excitatory type or an inhibitory type. Another way of stating this is that adrenergic drugs (including noradrenaline) are able to act either as excitatory or inhibitory ligands at adrenergic receptors.

Equally importantly, some direct-acting adrenoceptor blocking drugs bind to adrenergic receptors to attenuate or block the function of these receptors (that would normally result from their interaction with either adrenaline or noradrenaline) while other direct-acting adrenoceptor agonists (also known as adrenergic neuron blockers) augment the inhibitory action of the receptors that would also normally result from their interaction with noradrenaline.

In the CNS are two major medicines-relevant adrenoceptor-mediated activities – alpha$_1$-receptors are excitatory, while alpha$_2$-receptors are inhibitory. By current understanding, certain levels of brain noradrenaline pathways are needed as the basis for 'normal' balance and control of our state of (emotional) awareness and our ability to react and cope with life; inhibitory

pathways exert the opposite effect, including sedation and possible depression (see below).

A CNS beta$_2$-adrenergic blocking response was proposed as an explanation for depression or anxiety developing after use of some ophthalmic beta-blockers.[4] Both beta$_2$-blocker attenuation of excitatory adrenergic neurons, as well as presynaptic augmentation of dopaminergic neurons (see later) by beta-blockers, are possible CNS mechanisms.[5] While such effects could be attributed to substantial systemic absorption of beta-blocker eyedrops (Chapter 2), a lack of significant CNS absorption means that the beta-blockade is more likely to be peripheral.[6]

Drugs with indirect actions at catecholamine-mediated synapses in the CNS are used widely. These drugs should boost the adrenergic pathways and involve mechanisms that are a little more complex and involve both the synthesis, release, reuptake and metabolism of catecholamines. Legitimate stimulants include the CNS-active alpha- (and beta-?) receptor agonist ephedrine,[7] that is used widely to counter the sedative effects of antihistamines (e.g. in P Haymine, see below; Figure 3.2A). Some indirect-acting adrenergics produce mood-elevating effects (a CNS-sympathomimetic 'high', with peripheral effects)

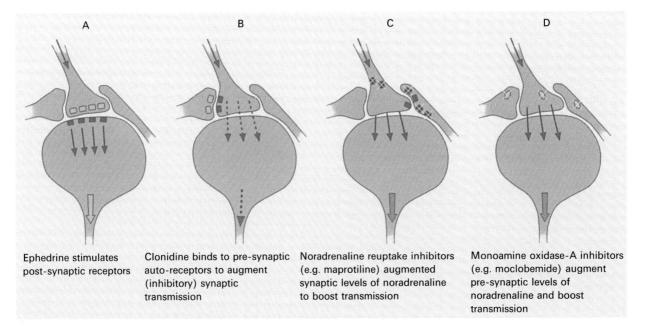

| A | B | C | D |
|---|---|---|---|
| Ephedrine stimulates post-synaptic receptors | Clonidine binds to pre-synaptic auto-receptors to augment (inhibitory) synaptic transmission | Noradrenaline reuptake inhibitors (e.g. maprotiline) augmented synaptic levels of noradrenaline to boost transmission | Monoamine oxidase-A inhibitors (e.g. moclobemide) augment pre-synaptic levels of noradrenaline and boost transmission |

**Figure 3.2**
*CNS adrenergic neurotransmission.*

both because they can promote unregulated neurotransmitter release from noradrenaline synapses and because they will activate the receptors for another catecholamine, serotonin.

Such use of cocaine or amphetamines can thus result in an overall uncontrolled sympathetic effect that results in agitation, elevated blood pressure, tachycardia, dilated pupils and hyperflexia or convulsions, and coma may also develop following abuse of this controlled drug (CD). Other 'amphetamines' include methylphenidate (CD Ritalin) which, although controversial in the UK, does have legitimate uses in attention deficit hyperactivity disorder (ADHD) management.[8] In contrast, the binding of clonidine to pre-synaptic alpha₂-receptors is considered to be able to block further noradrenaline release (Figure 3.2B). The pathway activity is attenuated with the net result that an inhibitory adrenergic signal emanates from the vasomotor centres.[9]

There are also a number of indirect-acting CNS-active adrenergics drugs that affect the catecholamine reuptake mechanisms.[10] These block the active transport of catecholamines back into the pre-synaptic terminals (Figure 3.2C) and include the tricyclic- (e.g. amitriptyline) and even tetracyclic- antidepressants (e.g. mianserin).

For each drug, the reuptake of one catecholamine may be blocked more than others. For example, noradrenaline reuptake is affected primarily by maprotiline (POM Ludiomil). Maprotiline is actually the metabolite of another drug called clomipramine (that is also clinically used, e.g. POM Anafranil) which exerts a slight preference to block the pre-synaptic reuptake of another CNS neurotransmitter called serotonin (see below). The administration of maprotiline will thus initially affect noradrenaline-mediated synapses and later affect serotonin-mediated synapses in the CNS. Such pro-drug effects are commonplace among CNS-neuroactive drugs. Newer drugs are considered to block re-uptake of serotonin much more than noradrenaline, and are known as serotonin-noradrenaline reuptake inhibitors or SNRIs, e.g. venlafaxine (POM Efexor).[11]

Some of these drugs (e.g. trimipramine, POM Surmontil), while generally affecting noradrenaline and serotonin reuptake, also have pronounced antimuscarinic (cholinergic-blocking) actions, producing

a sedating action on patients which makes them useful as sleep aids. As a result of both antidepressant and sedative effects, other tricyclic drugs (e.g. amitriptyline) can also be used to effect in the prophylactic management of migraine.[12]

After reuptake, inactivation is effected by monoamine oxidase (MAO) enzymes in the pre-synaptic terminal (Figure 3.2D). Such inhibition of the biotransformation raises pre-synaptic neurotransmitter levels and thus increases the frequency of possible synaptic transmission events. Another enzyme activity called catechol-O-methyl-transferase (COMT) is usually considered to be present within the synaptic cleft and plays some role in the biotransformation of catecholamines.

The enzyme monoamine oxidase should be well known to optometrists since concurrent administration of MAO inhibitors with large doses of eyedrops containing phenylephrine should be avoided.[13] Drugs such as phenelzine (e.g. POM Nardil) are MAO inhibitors and their use can be expected to boost brain catecholamine levels, providing a mood-elevating effect; the indications for use of this type of MAO inhibitor include depression. However, as the inactivation of noradrenaline is reduced, a general indirect sympathetic effect is produced in the CNS and elsewhere in the body, with the drug-mediated effect being indirect because the actual adrenergic receptors are not affected.

The dose of oral phenelzine should thus be carefully controlled to limit the extent of these sympathetic effects throughout the body. It is now known that there are two types of MAO localised at different nerve terminals in the CNS. The predominant enzyme activity is MAO-A and is associated with predominantly noradrenergic synapses, but there is a second type (MAO-B) at other brain locations.[14] Phenelzine is now recognised as a non-specific MAO inhibitor since it will inhibit both type A and type B forms of the enzyme.

More recently developed drugs are specific inhibitors of MAO type A.[15] These antidepressants are reversible inhibitors of monoamine oxidase A (RIMAs), e.g. moclobemide (POM Manerix). There is also a MAO type B inhibitor, selegiline (POM Eldepryl), which should boost synaptic dopamine (and noradrenaline) levels in patients with Parkinson's disease.[16] COMT inhibitors, such as entacapone (POM Comtess) are also used to boost peripheral

synapse dopamine and noradrenaline levels and can be useful in Parkinson's disease.[17]

Selegiline can also be considered as a pro-drug for serotonin receptors since it is biotransformed to amphetamines which then act at these receptors (see below).[18]

## Acetylcholine-mediated neurotransmission

In the CNS, a single cholinergic neurotransmitter exists, namely acetylcholine; it is not a catecholamine. The transmitter is present in many CNS pathways and at the ganglia linking the CNS with the parasympathetic branches of the autonomic nervous system (ANS). Acetylcholine or direct-acting cholinergic drugs bind directly to cholinergic receptors to augment their function and thus increase cholinergic synaptic activity.

Acetylcholine binds to CNS receptors (nicotinic and muscarinic) to activate pathways that determine our state of cognition and motor (muscle) coordination.[19] Acetylcholine can be released from pre-synaptic vesicles and bind to post-synaptic receptors to promote synaptic transmission. Acetylcholine is then inactivated by acetylcholinesterase or choline esterase enzymes, with the rate of this biotransformation being attenuated by acetylcholinesterase inhibitors (also known as 'anticholinesterases').

The inhibitors can be reversible or irreversible, to result in short- or long-term effects. These behave as indirect-acting cholinergic drugs because they do not bind to the cholinergic receptor, but will maintain synaptic levels of acetylcholine at higher levels for longer periods of time to augment synaptic transmission. As presently understood, there is no reuptake of acetylcholine similar to that for catecholamines.

The 'antimuscarinic' drugs (also known as anticholinergic drugs) are well known for their use as cycloplegic–mydriatics (e.g. tropicamide). However, other cholinergic-blocking drugs selectively act in the CNS to attenuate cholinergic functions and thus counteract (or even reverse) the actions that would be produced by acetylcholine.

To understand this selectivity, it should be noted that there are two general types of receptors that operate with acetylcholine

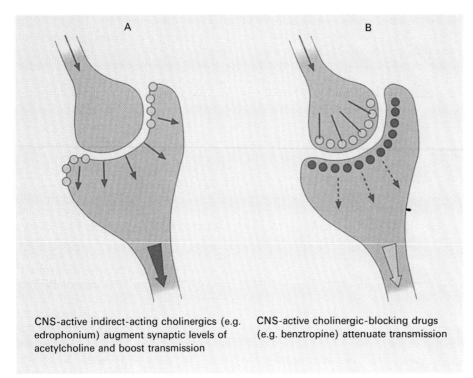

CNS-active indirect-acting cholinergics (e.g. edrophonium) augment synaptic levels of acetylcholine and boost transmission

CNS-active cholinergic-blocking drugs (e.g. benztropine) attenuate transmission

**Figure 3.3**
*CNS cholinergic neurotransmission.*

for the CNS. There are 'nicotinic' acetylcholine receptors that are located at discrete nerve bundles (nuclei) in the CNS and brainstem, and also at ganglia that serve both the sympathetic and parasympathetic branches of the ANS. All these will be affected diffusely by indirect-acting cholinergics. In addition, there are the muscarinic acetylcholine receptors located at discrete CNS nuclei as well as all end-plates in the parasympathetic branch of the ANS. Research over the past few years has shown that there are several subclasses of muscarinic cholinergic receptor ($m_1$, $m_2$, $m_3$ and $m_4$) but it remains controversial as to whether clinically used antimuscarinic drugs really do have receptor-selective action, or simply have preferential absorption into the CNS.[20]

Direct-acting cholinergics currently are not used intentionally as CNS-modifying agents,[21] while new indirect-acting cholinergics such as donepezil (POM Aricept) are for dementias typified by conditions such as Alzheimer's disease.[22] The idea behind such therapies is to boost those CNS pathways (Figure 3.3A) that are thought to be deteriorating in senile dementias such that some degree of normality is returned to our responsivity to normal life-style-related cues and stimuli and to improve short-term memory.

The downside of such drug use is that there is a risk of a parkinsonism-like condition (see below) being produced as an ADR. Other indirect-acting cholinergics such as edrophonium, not used for specific CNS-modulating effects, can be used temporarily to improve muscle tone, but more as intravenous or intramuscular injection as a test for myasthenia-like syndromes.[23] Edrophonium would be likely to be encountered only in a specialist hospital clinic (and actually may be prepared by a hospital pharmacy).

From the opposite perspective and with judicious monitoring of administration, CNS-active, cholinergic-blocking drugs can also be used to manage a relative excess of cholinergic activity (Figure 3.3B). This excess results from degeneration of dopamine-mediated pathways where the resultant condition is generally known as Parkinson's disease.[24]

Drugs such as benztropine (POM Cogentin) bind to select CNS-located muscarinic receptors in the extrapyramidal nuclei and produce a general sedating effect, attenuate hypersensitivity (in awareness that makes such patients tend to be overanxious) and should promote some reduction in uncontrolled motor activities.

Other drugs with cholinergic-blocking actions and which can cross the blood–brain barrier are also used widely to control our somatosensory systems to alleviate conditions such as nausea or dizziness (e.g. promazine, POM Sominex).

However, the binding of benztropine or other CNS-active cholinergic-blocking drugs to other poorly defined sites in the CNS can also alter our state of awareness such that hallucinations or similar effects develop.[25]

At high doses, any atropine-like drugs can cross the blood–brain barrier sufficiently to produce alterations in our state of awareness similar to benztropine, e.g. ophthalmic cyclopentolate or atropine.[3]

## Serotonin-mediated neurotransmission

Serotonin is another amine neurotransmitter that principally acts in the CNS, although serotonin-modulating drugs can have mood-elevating effects and vasoactive properties. The name serotonin has now largely replaced the use of other chemical names for this such as 5-hydroxytryptamine, although the receptor subtypes are still represented by the accepted abbreviation, 5-HT (see below).

Serotonin is considered to act at various excitatory nerve–nerve synapses in the CNS and brain and thus has some actions that are similar to noradrenaline. The serotonin pathways ascend from the brainstem through to the striatum and forebrain. In addition, portions of the cerebral vasculature are considered to be very sensitive to serotonin such that the relative intracranial blood flow compared with the extracranial blood vessels is regulated by serotonin levels.

Serotonin is stored in vesicles in nerve terminals and adjacent glial cells, and following its release it can bind to different receptor types known as 5-HT$_1$, 5-HT$_2$, 5-HT$_3$, 5-HT$_4$, etc, that have a number of subtypes as well. After dissociating from its receptors, serotonin is reabsorbed into the pre-synaptic terminals by a specific reuptake mechanism that can be blocked by a range of drugs. This reuptake terminates the serotoninergic neurotransmission, and some serotonin will be biotransformed by monoamine oxidase.

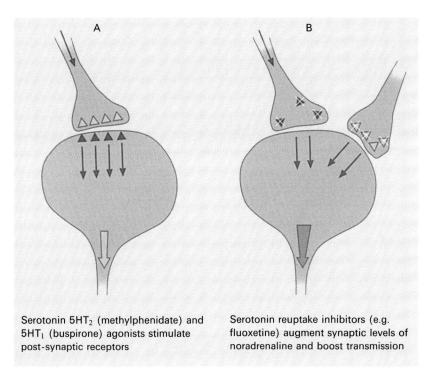

Serotonin 5HT$_2$ (methylphenidate) and 5HT$_1$ (buspirone) agonists stimulate post-synaptic receptors

Serotonin reuptake inhibitors (e.g. fluoxetine) augment synaptic levels of noradrenaline and boost transmission

**Figure 3.4**
*CNS serotoninergic neurotransmission.*

Overall, CNS-active serotoninergic drugs have become widely used in recent years, although direct-acting serotoninergic drugs have had limited clinical use. Hallucinogenic drugs, such as LSD, are considered able to bind to select 5-HT receptors to produce a CNS 'high'. Methylphenidate (oral POM Ritalin) is thought to act as an agonist at the same receptor,[8] probably 5-HT$_2$ (Figure 3.4A).

In the 1950s, amphetamines were used widely as appetite suppressants, which is an effect that perhaps results from their added actions at 5-HT$_2$ receptors. A lack of appetite suppression can cause substantial weight gain, which is an unwanted side-effect from the now less-used antimigraine drug methysergide (e.g. POM Deseril) that is thought also to bind to serotonin 5-HT$_2$ receptors.[12]

Drugs acting as stimulants of 5-HT$_1$ receptors (e.g. buspirone, POM BusPar) have limited use as anti-anxiety drugs.[26] However, it is the indirect-acting serotoninergic (serotonin-stimulating) drugs that have now become widely used as mood-elevators and antidepressants (Figure 3.4B). These include fluoxetine (e.g. POM Prozac), and sertraline (e.g. POM Lustral). These drugs are known as serotonin re-uptake inhibitors (SRIs) or selective serotonin reuptake inhibitors (SSRIs).[27]

Another CNS-active serotonin-modulating drug will also be encountered commonly in optometric practice because of the well-known association between migraine and eye symptoms. Sumatriptan (available as subcutaneous injectables, oral tablets and now as a nasal spray; POM Imigran) is a CNS-specific 5-HT$_1$ receptor agonist[28] that is believed to promote a general increase in cerebral blood flow to relieve migraine.[12] Similar effects can be expected from a selective 5-HT$_1$ agonist zolmitriptan (oral POM Zomig).

## Dopamine-mediated neurotransmission

Dopamine is another catecholamine that binds at many sites in the CNS where there are also noradrenaline-mediated synapses such that the 'activation' of inhibitory synapses can antagonise the excitatory effects of noradrenaline. Some dopamine pathways appear to mimic the cholinergic pathways.

The dopamine pathways arise in the upper portions of the brainstem and ascend to both the forebrain and the striatum areas, i.e. overlapping those regions served by serotonin. Alternatively, and concurrently, there can be further 'activation' of adrenergic synapses that are already inhibitory (i.e. alpha$_2$-adrenergic pathways).

Dopamine-mediated synapses also regulate synapses of other neurotransmitters, such as acetylcholine, so as to play a role in regulation of fine motor coordination.

Dopamine is released from pre-synaptic vesicles and will bind principally to post-synaptic D1 receptors (generally to initiate inhibitory responses).[7] In addition, the synaptic levels and release of the transmitter are regulated by pre-synaptic D2 and beta$_2$-receptor systems (another autoregulatory system).[7]

There is a reuptake mechanism for dopamine that is probably affected to some extent by other reuptake blocking drugs, and other drugs such as bupropion are being assessed as noradrenaline-dopamine reuptake inhibitors (Figure 3.5A).[29] Once reuptake has occurred, dopamine is metabolised by monoamine oxidase, especially MAO-B.

For patients with chronically suppressed dopaminergic systems (e.g. those with Parkinson's disease), direct-acting dopaminergics such as levodopa can be used to boost the contribution of dopaminergic pathways (Figure 3.5B) to control fine motor tremors and hypoactive rigidity since it raises the activity level of these dopamine-mediated inhibitory synapses.[24] Such 'activation' will suppress the relative excess of a CNS-originating cholinergic-parasympathetic system that ultimately causes the parkinsonian condition.

Levodopa is actually another pro-drug which is metabolised to dopamine. To maximise CNS effects, levodopa is usually co-administered with drugs such as carbidopa that reduce the peripheral biotransformation of levodopa to dopamine. Indirect-acting dopaminergics will also raise the level of some dopaminergic pathways (Figure 3.5C).

Drugs that act as inhibitors of MAO-B (e.g. selegiline, POM Eldepryl) will raise dopamine levels in pre-synaptic terminals to boost the contribution made by these inhibitory pathways on fine motor control;[24] selegiline also probably has some blocking actions on dopamine reuptake.

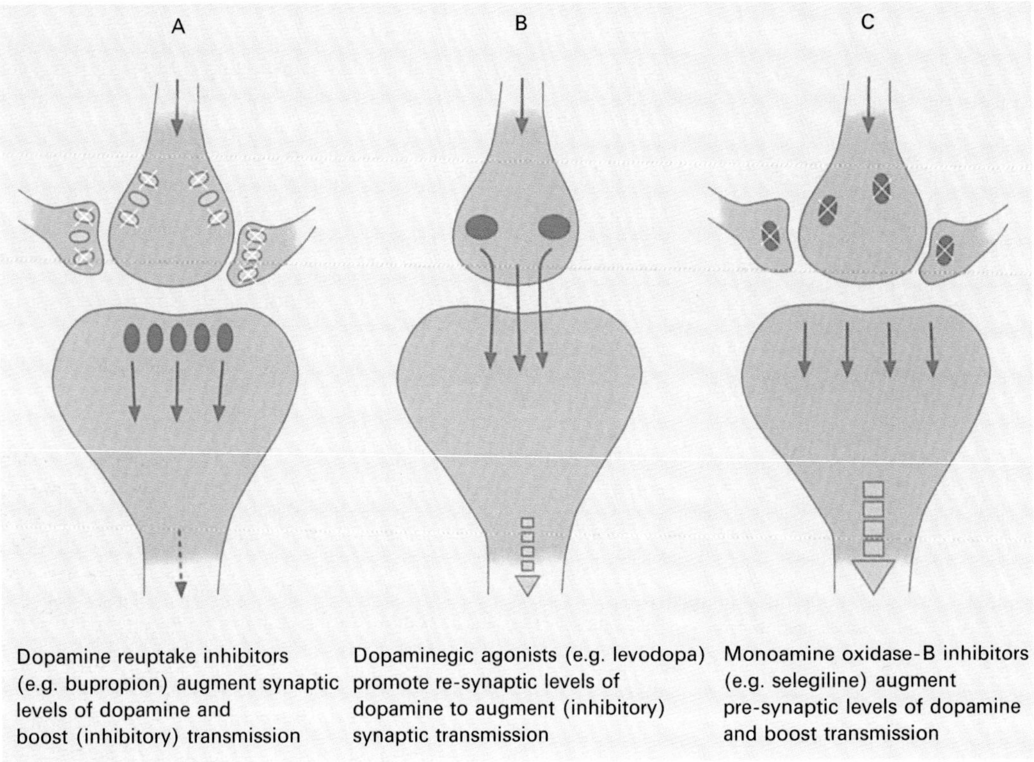

Dopamine reuptake inhibitors (e.g. bupropion) augment synaptic levels of dopamine and boost (inhibitory) transmission

Dopaminegic agonists (e.g. levodopa) promote re-synaptic levels of dopamine to augment (inhibitory) synaptic transmission

Monoamine oxidase-B inhibitors (e.g. selegiline) augment pre-synaptic levels of dopamine and boost transmission

**Figure 3.5**
*CNS dopaminergic neurotransmission.*

The neuroleptic or antipsychotic drugs (e.g. the phenothiazine-type drug chlorpromazine, POM Largactil) are now recognised as having substantial dopaminergic blocking effects and can calm individuals with psychoses and even delirium without necessarily sedating the patient.[30]

Psychoses have been considered generally to be the result of an over-reactive inhibitory dopaminergic system in the forebrain, and blockade by dopamine antagonists both counters such overreactivity and restores the balance of emotional (adrenergic) and cognitive functions (cholinergic).

The pathways by which such a balance is achieved appear complex since these drugs principally display high affinity binding to dopamine D2 pre-synaptic receptors and these seem to be located primarily on cholinergic neurons. Dopamine D2 receptor blockade at these sites results in increased activity (a disinhibition) of these pathways, since the D2 autoreceptor functions to reduce acetylcholine release.

Post-synaptic blockade of D2 receptors presumably reinforces such an effect to produce the cataleptic (calming) effect of

neuroleptics. Neuroleptics also have a range of effects at other receptors that are the most likely cause of side-effects, although a range of multireceptor neuroleptic drugs is now available that could have a lesser propensity for side-effects, e.g. risperidone (POM Risperdal, an antagonist for both 5-HT$_2$ and D2 receptors)[31] or buspirone (POM BusPar, acting as a D2 antagonist but 5-HT$_1$ agonist).

That the dopamine-mediated pathways play such a pivotal role in the functional interaction of CNS neuron types is aptly illustrated by the fact that a well-known and potentially very serious ADR from neuroleptic therapy is the induction of a parkinsonian condition;[30] this iatrogenic effect is then managed through the use of CNS-active cholinergic blocking drugs (see above).

## GABA-mediated neurotransmission

Gamma-aminobutyric acid (GABA) is largely a CNS-based neurotransmitter found in both nerves and glial cells, but it is

becoming increasingly apparent that there are numerous peripheral sites with GABA receptors.[32] The organisation of GABA-ergic synapses and their localisation is less well understood but generally is believed to be concentrated in the forebrain areas, especially the thalamus and cortex. It can only be generalised that the release of GABA will result in binding to postsynaptic receptors of the inhibitory type.

The CNS appears to contain a principal GABA receptor type A [GABA(A)] but a GABA(B) receptor is also now known. GABA reuptake occurs, but GABA biotransformation occurs via the action of GABA transaminase.

GABA-modulating drugs are often known as hypnotics because of their propensity, at high dose, to induce substantial sedation. GABA, working via GABA(A) receptors, has a distinct role in regulating our state of awareness and its overall role is to modulate the excitatory pathways operated through noradrenaline or serotonin. Hypoactivity in GABA-regulated pathways leads to states of over-reaction to stimulation and stress, and especially in our ability to relax and sleep, and thus the

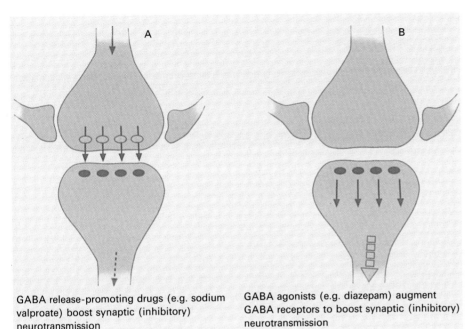

GABA release-promoting drugs (e.g. sodium valproate) boost synaptic (inhibitory) neurotransmission

GABA agonists (e.g. diazepam) augment GABA receptors to boost synaptic (inhibitory) neurotransmission

**Figure 3.6**
*CNS GABA-ergic neurotransmission.*

use of GABA-ergic drugs to promote somnolence and manage parasomnias.

The drugs that are used widely, however, clinically directly bind to GABA(A) receptors, and act as agonists to boost inhibitory pathways.[33] A GABA analogue, gabapentin (POM Neurontin), or a drug that promotes release of GABA (sodium valproate, POM Convulex), are other direct and indirect-acting GABA-mimetics (Figure 3.6A). An alternative indirect mechanism is the use of drugs that boost GABA levels by inhibiting GABA biotransformation, e.g. vigabatrin (POM Sabitril).[34] These drugs may also have some GABA-mimetic actions, just as gabapentin may have some inhibitory action on GABA transaminase. These drugs are also known as CNS depressants because they boost inhibitory pathways.

Other CNS depressants include the benzodiazepines (e.g. diazepam; POM Valium), use of which has now largely replaced the use of barbiturates (e.g. amylobarbitone; CD Amytal) that act on the same receptor-synapse system (Figure 3.6B). Benzodiazepines are used widely to manage anxiety, as sleep aids (e.g. nitrazepam, POM Mogodon) and as pre-surgery sedatives and relaxants.[33] Barbiturates (e.g. phenobarbitone, CD) can still be used to manage refractory epilepsy but benzodiazepines

(e.g. clonazepam, POM Rivotril) or sodium valproate are more widely used for epilepsy.[35]

An overdose, deep sleep or even a coma can be induced with all these drugs. Ethanol (ethyl alcohol) also acts as a CNS depressant (i.e. boosting inhibitory pathways) by augmenting the activity of GABA receptors and any combinations of ethanol with barbiturates or benzodiazepines can be fatal. A GABA(B) receptor agonist is baclofen (POM Lioresal), used to counter the effects of a range of motoneuron disorders,[36] including following strokes.

## Histamine-mediated neurotransmission

Histamine is still a relatively poorly understood bioactive substance, especially in terms of neurological functions,[37] although histamine-blocking drugs ('antihistamines') are very widely used. Select histamine blocking (e.g. hydroxyzine, oral POM Atarax) can be used effectively as anti-anxiety drugs because of their sedative effects.

Other select histamine blocking drugs, such as cyclizine, can be used for migraine (e.g. POM Migril) or for nausea (e.g. POM

Valoid), while both promazine (POM Sominex) and diphenhydramine (P Nytol) also exert substantial sedative effects[37,38] and are known to cross readily the blood–brain barrier.[20]

While action at any of the other CNS synapses (e.g. dopaminergic and cholinergic synapses for promazine) may be a cause of such effects, they can all be used to good effect to control nausea and travel sickness,[38] as well as promote sleep.

## Summary of medications for the CNS and their use

The six principal CNS neurotransmitters reviewed in this chapter are only part of the story, for a range of other neuroactive substances (especially bioactive peptides) are also produced and released in the CNS to control our perception and somatosensory systems, including that of pain.

The vasculature external to and within the CNS is also substantially regulated by a range of vasoactive substances beyond adrenaline, serotonin, and histamine and include nitric oxide and prostaglandins. The activity of the latter compounds, coupled with the cholinergic systems are linked to the central processing of pain by mechanisms that include the actions of bioactive peptides (such as substance P) and the opiate receptors (that mediate the actions of morphine and related drugs).

Overall, however, a vast range of CNS-active drugs are common prescription medications in the population at large to manage blood pressure, depression, dementias, anxiety, migraine, motoneuron disorders, alimentary tract dysfunction, schizophrenia, sleep disorders, epilepsy and nausea.

## General impact of CNS drugs on the eye and vision

The very nature of many of the conditions than can be managed effectively by CNS-active drugs means some patients may find it difficult to divulge their history of such medication usage to their optometrist, so extra vigilance in taking a medications history is important.

The reason for stressing the importance of having complete details of these diverse medications is because they can have subtle or profound effects on the eye and vision. Of all the ADR listings relevant to the eye that can be found in various directories such as the *Monthly Index of Medical Specialities* (Chapter 1), at least one in five relates to CNS-active drugs affecting oculomotor coordination, eye movements or vision in a non-specified manner.

It is uncommon for any of these ADRs to be detailed specifically but the key words are not only blurred vision but also 'visual disturbances', 'CNS disturbances' or 'extrapyramidal reactions'. Where 'anticholinergic effects' are listed as ADRs or precautions, there are obviously potential effects on most parts of the eye including vision *per se*.[39]

As noted earlier, all such drugs potentially could interact with sympathomimetic or parasympatholytic drugs used in therapies for the eye. With repeated use, the chance of unwanted iatrogenic events increases, so increased vigilance to avoid such drug–drug interactions is not only appropriate but would constitute safe practice.

# References

1 O'Conner Davies PH, Hopkins GA, Pearson RM (1989) *The Actions and Uses of Ophthalmic Drugs*, 3rd edn. Butterworths, London.

2 Vale J, Cox B (1978) *Drugs and the Eye*. Butterworths, London.

3 Jarvinen K, Jarvinel T, Urtti A (1995) Ocular absorption following topical delivery. *Adv Drug Delivery Rev* **16**: 3–19.

4 Duch S, Duch C, Pasto L *et al.* (1992) Changes in depressive status associated with topical beta-blockers. *Int Ophthalmol* **16**: 331–335.

5 Misu Y, Goshima Y (1993) Is L-dopa an endogenous neurotransmitter? *Trends Pharmacol Sci* **14**: 119–123.

6 Tyrer P (1992) Anxiolytics not acting at the benzodiazepine receptor: beta blockers. *Progr Neuro-Psychopharmacol Biol-Psychiat* **6**: 17–26.

7 Kuitunen T, Karkkainen S, Ylitalo P (1984) Comparison of the acute physical and mental effects of ephedrine, fenfluramine, phentermine and prolintane. *Meth Find Exp Clin Pharmacol* **6**: 265–270.

8 Nigg JT, Swanson JM, Hinshaw SP (1997) Covert visual spatial attention in boys with atention deficit hyperactivity disorder: lateral effects, methylphenidate response and results for parents. *Neuropsychologia* **35**: 165–176.

9 Houston MC (1981) Clonidine hydrochloride: review of pharmacologic and clinical aspects. *Progr Cardiovasc Dis* **23**: 337–349.

10 Rudnick G, Clark J (1993) From synapse to vesicle: the reuptake and storage of biogenic amine neurotransmitters. *Biochim Biophys Acta* **1144**: 249–263.

11 Scott MA, Shelton PS, Gattis W (1996) Therapeutic options for treating major depression, and the role of venlafaxine. *Pharmacotherapy* **16**: 352–365.

12 Doughty MJ, Lyle WM (1995) Medications used to prevent migraine headaches and their potential ocular adverse effects. *Optom Vis Sci* **72**: 879–891.

13 Gimpel G, Doughty MJ, Lyle MW (1994) Large sample study of the effects of phenylephrine 2.5% eyedrops on the amplitude of accommodation in man. *Ophthal Physiol Opt* **14**: 123–128.

14 Berry MD, Juorio AV, Paterson IA (1994) The functional role of monoamine oxidases A and B in the mammalian central nervous system. *Prog Neurobiol* **42**: 375–391.

15 Buller R (1995) Reversible inhibitors of monoamine oxidase A in anxiety disorders. *Clin Neuropharmacol* **18** (S-2): S38–S44.

16 Oreland L (1991) Monoamine oxidase, dopamine and Parkinson's disease. *Acta Neurol Scand* **84** (suppl 136): 60 65.

17 Ruottinen HM, Rinne UK (1996) Effect of one month's treatment with peripherally acting catechol-O-methyltransferase inhibitor, entacapone, on pharmacokinetics and motor response to levodopa in advanced parkinsonian patients. *Clin Neuropharmacol* **19**: 222–233.

18 Reynolds GP, Elsworth K, Blau M *et al.* (1978) Deprenyl is metabolized to methamphetamine and amphetamine in man. *Br J Clin Pharmacol* **6**: 542–544.

19 Palacios JM, Boddeke HWGM, Pombo-Villar E (1991) Cholinergic neuropharmacology: an update. *Acta Psychiatr Scand* (suppl 266): 27–33.

20 Tamai I, Tsuji A (1996) Drug delivery through the blood-brain barrier. *Adv Drug Delivery* **19**: 401–424.

21 Cutler NR, Sramek JJ (1995) Muscarinic M(1)-receptor agonists – potential in the treatment of Alzheimer's disease. *CNS Drugs* **3**: 467–481.

22 Schneider LS, Tariot PN (1994) Emerging drugs for Alzheimer's disease. Mechanisms of action and prospects for cognitive enhancing medications. *Med Clin N America* **78**: 911–934.

23 Oh SJ, Cho HK (1990) Endrophonium responsiveness not necessarily diagnostic of myasthenia gravis. *Muscle Nerve* **13**: 187–191.

24 Mizuno Y, Mori H, Kondo T (1994) Practical guidelines for the drug-treatment of Parkinson's disease. *CNS Drugs* **1**: 410–426.

25 Marken PA, Stoner SC, Bunker MT (1996) Anticholinergic drug abuse and misuse – epidemiology and therapeutic implications. *CNS Drugs* **5**: 190–199.

26 Taylor DP, Moon SL (1991) Buspirone and related compounds as alternative anxiolytics. *Neuropeptides* **19** (suppl): 15–19.

27 Åsberg M, Mårtensson B (1993) Serotonin selective antidepressant drugs: past, present, future. *Clin Neuropharmacol* **16** (S-3): S32–S44.

28 Dechant KL, Clissold SP (1992) Sumatriptan. A review of its pharmacodynamic and pharmacokinetic properties, and therapeutic efficacy in the acute treatment of migraine and cluster headache. *Drugs* **43**: 776–798.

29 Preskorn SH (1994) Antidepressant drug selection: criteria and options. *J Clin Psychiatry* **55** (suppl A): 6–22.

30 Gershanik OS (1994) Drug-induced parkinsonism in the aged. Recognition and prevention. *Drugs Aging* **5**: 127–132.

31 He H, Richardson JS (1995) A pharmacological, pharmacokinetic and clinical overview of risperidone, a new antipsychotic that blocks serotonin 5-HT2 and dopamine D2 receptors. *Int Clin Psychopharmacol* **10**: 19–30.

32 Möhler H (1992) GABAergic synaptic transmission. Regulation by drugs. *Drug Res* **42**: 211–214.

33 Bartholini G (1985) GABA receptor agonists: pharmacological spectrum

and therapeutic actions. *Med Res Rev* **5**: 55–75.

34 French LA (1999) Vigabatrin. *Epilepsia* **40** (suppl 5): S11–S16.

35 Heller AJ, Chesterman P, Elwes RDC *et al.* (1995) Phenobarbitone, phenytoin, carbamazepine, or sodium valproate for newly diagnosed adult epilepsy: a randomised comparative monotherapy trial. *J Neurol Neurosurg Psychiat* **58**: 44–50.

36 Misgeld U, Bijak M, Jarolimek W (1995) A physiological role for GABA(B) receptors and the effects of baclofen in the mammalian central nervous system. *Prog Neurobiol* **46**: 423–462.

37 Leurs R, Smit MJ, Timmerman H (1995) Molecular pharmacological aspects of histamine receptors. *Pharmacol Therap* **3**: 413–463.

38 Rascol O, Hain TC, Brefel C *et al.* (1995) Antivertigo medications and drug-induced vertigo. A pharmacological review. *Drugs* **50**: 777–791.

39 Doughty MJ (1999) The ocular side effects of CNS-acting drugs. *Optician* **218**: 17–26.

# 4

# Ophthalmic pharmaceuticals, their formulation and use

Legislation pertaining to pharmaceutical formulation
Basic ingredients of ophthalmic pharmaceuticals
Properties of different constituents of ophthalmic pharmaceuticals
Vehicles
Buffers
Preservatives
Stabilisers

## Introduction

Solutions (eyedrops), gels and ointments designated for external ophthalmic use constitute a very special group of pharmaceuticals. These products are made available to both health care professionals and the public at large as a result of being marketed by registered companies.

The principal mode of supply is through a registered pharmacist, although specifically designated products are available through retail outlets such as supermarkets (general sales list – GSL – products).

Another approved route for optometrists, other than via pharmacists, is by direct supply of designated pharmaceuticals and other non-medicinal products including mail-order supply.[1-3]

Pharmaceuticals legitimately marketed through pharmacists have to be dispensed in an approved form and container which should have some details of what is in the product in terms of the actual 'active' ingredient as based upon certain formulation guidelines. The pharmaceutical companies are also encouraged to give some details of the other ingredients, either by acknowledging a certain

formulation guideline, or by giving specific details.

It is the goal of this chapter to explain why different types of formulations of ophthalmic pharmaceuticals are available in the UK and why knowledge of these is an important step to selecting and using pharmaceuticals in primary eye care. There is also a need to come to terms with what the 'small print' on each product is meant to communicate to either the optometrist or the end-point user.

The preparation of solutions, ointments or gels intended for presentation to the external eye (in the UK) should always be done by the laboratory in a registered pharmaceutical company or at a government-approved pharmacy service. Should practitioners consider *ad hoc* formulation (e.g. by mixing commercially available ophthalmic products), it has to be stressed that the potential risks in using such a product far outweigh the potential benefit.

An increasing number of ophthalmic 'pharmaceuticals' are becoming available either as contact lens-related products (and should carry a $C\epsilon$ label; Chapter 1) or even non-medicinal products, essentially as cosmetics or beauty aids.

## Ophthalmic pharmaceutical product types

### Current perspectives

Optometrists are already familiar with the availability of several ophthalmic solutions in single-use containers, i.e. the Minims line of products which consists of containers made from clear plastic with a snap-off cap (see Figure 4.1). Such products are ideal for routine diagnostic drugs such as tropicamide 0.5 or 1%. These types of products contain a drug dissolved in a sterile aqueous solution, the details of which are generally not provided with the products.

These 'single-use' or 'unit-dose' products should deliver a drop size of approximately 30 μl.[4] While the containers can hold up to seven drops of a drug solution, they are not designated for multiple use under any circumstances.

Such single-use containers of mydriatics could be considered as ideal for an optometric practice since relatively small-sized batches can be purchased (i.e. a box of 20 units) and could probably be used before the expiry date (stamped on the outside packaging).

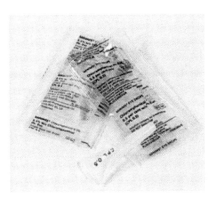

**Figure 4.1**
*MINIMS® single dose products.*

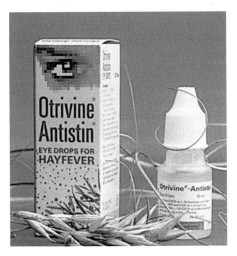

**Figure 4.2**
*Clear plastic bottles for multiple use.*

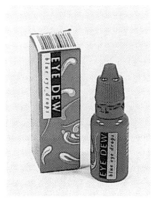

**Figure 4.3**
*Coloured opaque plastic bottles for multiple use.*

In other cases, the availability of diagnostic drugs such as proxymetacaine (proparacaine) or 0.5% rose bengal 1% in single-use containers serves an additional advantage because the product is inherently unstable and has a shorter shelf life and usage life when dispensed in a larger 5 ml bottle.

While such unit-dose containers have the advantage of a generally greater stability because they are sealed and for single-use only, they should still be stored according to manufacturers' instructions. Such instructions in the UK generally advise storage temperatures of between 8°C and 25°C (unless specifically detailed otherwise) and avoiding prolonged exposure to light.

The latter recommendation can be met easily by keeping unit-dose products in the cardboard carton in which they were supplied. It is especially important both because the Minims container is largely transparent to light and some of the ingredients, e.g. topical ocular anaesthetics, are known to be relatively unstable to light, especially when kept at warmer temperatures.

Keeping Minims products in their correct and original cartons should also reduce the risk of error in dispensing.

Optometrists are also familiar with the use of ophthalmic wafers, marketed in sterile external packaging for single use only, and where the drug is impregnated into the pharmaceutical form, e.g. fluorescein-impregnated strips for diagnostic use.

A limited number of therapeutic drugs are also available in unit-dose form.

Optometrists have the right to use, sell or otherwise supply designated pharmaceuticals of these types (e.g. chloramphenicol 0.5% eyedrops, Figure 4.1) in the course of their professional activity and in an emergency.[5] It should be noted that such a solution of chloramphenicol has a very slight yellow coloration because of the constituent chemical properties of the drug in solution. As the drug solution is not very stable, such products should be checked before use for any significant departure from this colour. According to manufacturers' instructions, the pharmaceutical should be stored at 4°C (i.e. in a normal refrigerator) and should not be left lying around at room temperature.

Should small quantities of the pharmaceutical be dispensed to a patient for emergency use, it is a good idea to check that the supply was in fact used at the time of follow-up or that the patient be asked to return any unused containers of the drug to reduce the chance of later usage of spoiled products.

**The multiple-use product in regular use**

Most ophthalmic pharmaceuticals are not supplied in unit-dose containers but are in multiple-dose bottles for repeated use by practitioners or patients, and now contain solutions of drugs specially formulated to be suitable for multiple use.

The containers are made of plastic and generally have a 5, 10 or 15 ml capacity. The plastic bottles for these P products have screw caps that cover a specially designed dropper tip which should dispense reliably one drop at a time on gentle pressure being applied to the bottle.

Usually these days the plastic for the bottles is an opaque white since this limits the light levels that the pharmaceutical may be exposed to during the course of normal use.

Such consideration of light sensitivity is important since certain drug solutions, while colourless at formulation, can discolour as a result of long-term exposure to light and oxygen. Examples here would include the adrenergic ophthalmic decongestant–antihistamine drug combinations (e.g. P Otrivine–Antistin, Figure 4.2) or antiglaucoma drugs such as adrenaline (see later).

Some other P products containing decongestants such as naphazoline are supplied in coloured plastic bottles (e.g. P Eye-Dew Blue, Figure 4.3) where the decongestant solution in this example also contains a dye called Brilliant Blue FCF. This is a British Pharmacopoeia-approved colorant for ophthalmic pharmaceuticals. As with other blue dyes, such as methylene blue,[6,7] the presence of a thin film of Brilliant Blue solution across the conjunctiva should serve to promote cosmesis, i.e. an improved appearance to a slightly reddened congested conjunctiva.

Other commonly used multi-use ophthalmic pharmaceuticals include the range of artificial tear products available as P products (e.g. P Liquifilm Tears, Figure 4.4) in multiple-use bottles for general use. Such products, as almost all other multiple-use products in this category, contain preservatives such as benzalkonium chloride or chlorbutanol.[8]

Despite the sometimes vociferate adverse press on the damaging effects of such

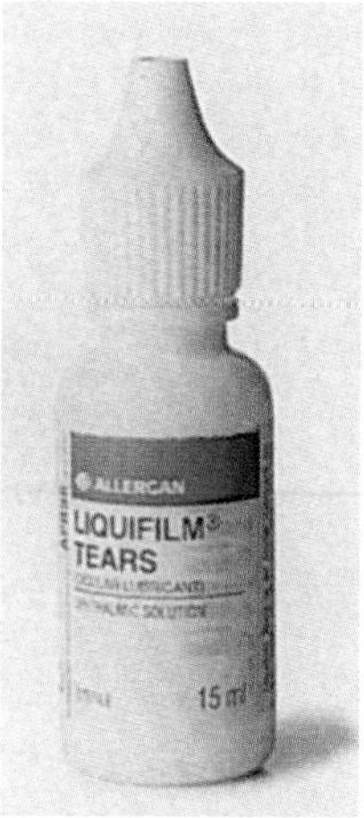

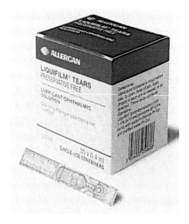

**Figure 4.4**
*Opaque plastic bottles for multiple use.*

**Figure 4.5**
*Preservative-free unit dose products for
therapeutic use.*

ingredients on the ocular surface, the fact
that very few adverse reaction reports are
filed on the use of such pharmaceuticals
surely argues against there being a hazard
or even a significant risk. However, if a
patient is perceived to be at risk from the development of a toxic conjunctivitis or keratitis consequent to the repeated exposure of
the surface of the eye to a preservative-containing solution, then special unit-dose formulations of some artificial tears are
available (e.g. Liquifilm Tears PF, Figure
4.5).

Such products are much more expensive
than multi-use bottles and generally will
not be supplied direct to customers by pharmacists, but rather through practitioners
for use by patients such as those with a

chronic but uncomplicated dry-eye history
who require frequent use of such products.

A useful guideline for what constitutes
frequent use would be more than six times
a day, although this concept does not
appear to have been substantiated by
detailed research.[7,8]

Relevant also to the use of preservative-
containing products is concurrent soft
(hydrogel) contact lens wear and whether
this constitutes an additional hazard to the
patient.[7,9] It has become increasingly
common place for ophthalmic pharmaceutical listings to include a contraindication
(C/I) for (soft) contact lenses on the basis of
largely unsubstantiated claims that the
lens matrix could act as a significant reservoir for the preservatives to promote a
toxic keratitis.[7]

The fact that such solutions have been
used widely concurrently with bandage
contact lenses in the very eyes that might
be considered at risk because a compromised epithelium is present surely argues
for the C/I to be reworded as a cautionary
note. Practitioners should always be on the
alert for the potential of ocular surface complications if a preservative-containing eyedrop is repeatedly used concurrent with
contact lens wear. Certain GSL or contact-
lens-wear-related products now carry the
warning on the label of 'do not use while or
immediately before wearing contact
lenses' and this seems a more useful guideline.[10] The 'immediately before' can be
translated into practical use as 5
minutes.[10,11]

The last type of ophthalmic solution in
widespread use is that of the astringent.
Such products contain chemicals such as
witch hazel (watery extracts of *Hamamelis*)
which are recognised as having additional
cleansing actions to the use of saline
alone[1,7,12] (e.g. P Optrex Eye Lotion, Figure
4.6). Such products are generally supplied
with an eye bath cup to facilitate effective
cleansing of the external eye.

## Towards the routine use of multi-use ophthalmic pharmaceuticals and the rationale behind their formulation

In the routine provision of primary eye
care, multi-use ophthalmic products will
generally be the standard type of pharmaceutical used both on the basis of economics
and convenience. There are a number of
important characteristics of multi-use
products that deserve consideration.

All ophthalmic pharmaceuticals have to

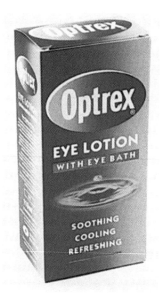

**Figure 4.6**
*Eye lotions containing an astringent.*

be sterile at the time they are dispensed,
and should be prepared in such a way so as
to maintain that sterility for their period of
recommended use.

The importance of sterilisation of pharmaceutical products designated for application to the external eye has long been
recognised.[13] The requirement for sterility
goes beyond simply considering whether
the solution is free of microorganisms,
since the ophthalmic solution, suspension,
ointment or gel has to be prepared from ingredients that are ultra-pure and that are
sterilised in such a way so as to generate
no products from the sterilisation process,
i.e. be pyrogen-free.[14,15]

All of the products should also meet very
strict requirements on particulates, e.g.
less than $0.22\ \mu m$ in size for standard types
of eyedrops. Without such quality
controls, the resultant product could prove
to be irritating to the human eye and/or
elicit some form of allergic reaction. Therefore, all ophthalmic pharmaceuticals have
to be manufactured following specific
guidelines and quality control measures,
and this applies to whether their ingredients or formulation is apparently simple or
complex.

Other important points relating to each
and every multidose ophthalmic pharmaceutical reflect the expected usage. Rather
than having a unit-dose container that is
opened once, one now has a container that
is going to be opened and closed repeatedly

under a range of environments in terms of temperature, humidity, pathogen levels and particulates.

As with a unit-dose pharmaceutical, the shelf life of a multi-use product is dictated by the expiry date stamped on the container. However, the multi-use pharmaceutical also has a usage life which is the period of time in which the opened multi-use pharmaceutical should be used after opening; a generally accepted guideline for the UK is that all such containers should be discarded one month after opening (see later).

Unit-dose ophthalmic pharmaceuticals for diagnostic purposes may be considered as the ideal when their use is occasional and irregular. However, since the routine pupil dilation of patients, especially first-time patients and those aged over 40 years, should become the acceptable standard of practice for all primary eye care, the selection of multi-use products is desirable in terms of efficiency and cost. Some such preparations are available as brand-name products (e.g. tropicamide, POM Mydriacyl, Figure 4.7).

Like unit-dose formulations, the multi-use containers for such products will usually list the minimal details of the ingredients, in this case it is stated to be 'tropicamide 1.0% in a sterile ophthalmic solution'. The packaging elaborates on this by stating 'tropicamide 1.0% BP, preservative benzalkonium chloride Ph. Eur. 0.01%'. An ABPI Compendium of Data Sheets (1997 edition, p. 22) could state that the 'presentation' of the pharmaceuti-

cal is as a sterile, clear, colourless solution'. The small print on the bottle states that the product should be stored between 8°C and 25°C and that it should be protected from light. The ABPI directs one to store these eyedrops in a cool place, additionally noting that they should not be refrigerated and should be kept away from direct sunlight. Such descriptors and the place they are found is changing however. In the 1999/2000 edition of the ABPI, (p. 32) exactly the same pharmaceutical is listed as 'sterile eye drops ...' with no mention of whether it is a clear, colourless solution! The storage guidelines have also been revised slightly to '... not exceeding 25°C', and (presumably by implication, since it also says 'do not refrigerate') the lower limit is unspecified but is presumably 4°C.

On consultation of these and other listings, it should be evident that there is unfortunately no standardisation of the information, and other major pharmaceutical directories can include slightly different details even of the same brand product. The issue here, however, is what this information means, why it is important and what might be encountered in different products. Consideration of each product is important for no two products are identical.

The drug concentration on the tropicamide eye drops (Figure 4.7) is specified to be 1.0%, which by implication is in weight/volume units, i.e. 1 g/100 ml of eye-drop solution. As a rough guideline, each ml of eyedrops thus contains 10 mg of tropicamide and this way of presenting the concentration can be found on some ophthalmic drugs (e.g. the quantity of trimethoprim in POM Polytrim, see Figure 4.19).

The accuracy of the formulation can be expected to be within ±10%, i.e. the concentration in this example should be between 0.9 and 1.1% at the time the product was dispensed, and this concentration should be maintained until the expiration date and also throughout the period of recommended use of the pharmaceutical.

The actual volume of a single eyedrop is not fixed since different dropper tips deliver 25 to 50 µl,[4,12] but a drop of 30 µl of a 1.0% solution would nominally contain 0.6 mg of the active ingredient. Thus the dose of the drug in each eyedrop (tropicamide in this example) that initially would be delivered to the surface of the eye is unambiguous; ambiguity in dosing with ophthalmic pharmaceuticals is the result

of essentially useless instructions such as 'instil eye drops into the affected eye when required'. For effective and safe delivery of ophthalmic drugs, the number of drops, and the frequency of eyedrop usage should be stipulated (Chapter 1).

That there can be reasonable reliance on the expected dose in each drop of the solution can be derived from the BP designation for the active drug on this pharmaceutical, or the 'Ph Eur' on the preservative (see Figure 4.1) or 'BPC' (see Figure 4.22). For example, the 'BP' stands for British Pharmacopoeia, which contains detailed recommendations, principally directed at the manufacturers and hospital pharmacies, on how to prepare a particular type of eyedrop or ointment, etc. The 'Ph Eur' designation also indicates that the preservative, benzalkonium chloride, meets with specific purity guidelines, for benzalkonium chloride is not a single chemical substance.

In a busy practice, such multi-use bottles of mydriatics should still be discarded on a monthly basis even though they are preserved and stabilised. Overall, detailed formulation information for ophthalmic pharmaceuticals was once considered important for optometrists,[16] but really has little relevance nowadays for the provision of primary eye care medicines.

## The characteristics of therapeutic ophthalmic pharmaceuticals

Multi-use eye drop products containing nothing other than sodium chloride (P Sodium Chloride, Figure 4.8) are available

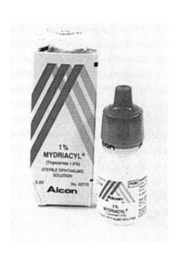

**Figure 4.7**
*Multi-use products containing drugs for diagnostic use.*

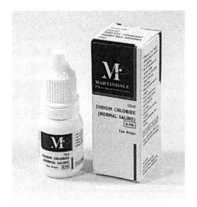

**Figure 4.8**
*Normal saline (sodium chloride) eyedrops.*

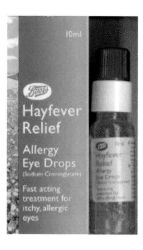

**Figure 4.9**
*Generic ophthalmic products for high street retail.*

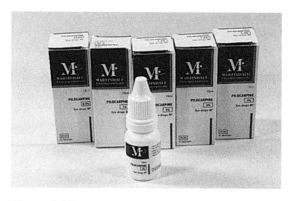

**Figure 4.10**
*Generic ophthalmic product line.*

as generics, which may need to be specially requested from a pharmacist. The designation of 'normal saline' can be taken as meaning that the concentration of sodium chloride (NaCl) is close to 0.9% w/v, and should not be uncomfortable to the human eye.[17] Such multi-use bottles, even if only of saline, will still contain a preservative such as benzalkonium chloride.

In common with many multi-use eye-drop products, such solutions are likely to be unbuffered (or contain just small quantities of pH-buffering chemicals) but could have very small quantities of acid (usually HCl) or alkali (usually NaOH) added to adjust the pH to be close to 7.0. The pH adjustment is important since it is likely that slightly acid (pH 6.0–6.5) eyedrops will elicit a transient stinging sensation while more neutral pH solutions will elicit a lesser effect.[18,19] More alkaline (pH 7.5–8.5) eyedrops can be expected to produce some mild discomfort. It might be argued therefore that all eyedrops should have a pH of between 6.5 and 7.5, but this is simply not practical. Many commonly used ophthalmic drugs need to be formulated in slightly acidic (e.g. topical ocular anaesthetics) or moderately acidic (pH 5.5–6.0) solutions (e.g. ophthalmic phenylephrine and some anti-microbials),[7,14] but even some artificial tear products containing polyvinyl alcohol (e.g. P Sno-Tears) may also be moderately acidic.

All such acidic eyedrops will almost invariably elicit a marked but transient stinging sensation and precipitate reflex tearing, but should not normally have any

significant adverse effects on the ocular surface since the pH film usually will be rapidly restored to its original level as a result of normal washout (Chapter 2) and the natural buffering capacity of the human tears.[20]

For a number of ophthalmic products, the commonly used pharmaceuticals directories (e.g. *MIMS* and the *BNF*) will list a brand-name product but not any generic equivalents. Some generic products can be found in the *BNF* but the manufacturers or distributors of such generic products can change even on a month-by-month basis.

There are several aspects of generics that need to be considered. First, the availability of a branded product does not mean that there is a generic equivalent. Secondly, a generic can only be marketed if there are no regulatory limits preventing it competing with the branded product. Thirdly, a generic equivalent must be able to compete effectively for a market share concurrently with the branded product, or even other generics.

It is therefore likely that proportionately more generics will be used in a hospital eye clinic than in a high-street practice simply because the larger volume sales can be expected to drive the already-competitive prices of the generics even lower. However, there are other types of 'generics' available through high-street retail markets, e.g. (Boots) P Hypromellose or P Hayfever Relief Allergy Eye Drops (containing sodium cromoglycate 2%). The unusual presentation bottle type and cap should be noted for the latter product (Figure 4.9).

Potentially to confuse things, it needs to be noted that such anticipated large volume sales can also mean that the manufacturer of a brand-name product will then

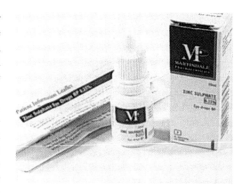

**Figure 4.11**
*Generic ophthalmic products as replacements for brand-name products.*

produce its own 'generic' equivalent for hospital use after the patent protection period for its branded product has expired, e.g. timolol eyedrops marketed both as POM Timoptol and as generic POM Timolol Eye Drops, or pilocarpine eyedrops marketed as POM IsoptoCarpine and POM Pilocarpine Eye Drops (Figure 4.10).

Lastly, it is important to note that generic products can persist long after a brand-name product has disappeared from the market. Multiple-use bottles of saline eyedrops (see Figure 4.8) are one such example and another is zinc sulphate eyedrops (Figure 4.11). Zinc sulphate eyedrops and solutions have soothing, astringent and mild bacteriostatic actions with several products being sold in the past.[1] With such an eyedrop being used for many years, there is no longer any need for a company to recoup the costs of development, and the only viable product is a generic, although it still has to meet specific formulation requirements. This is

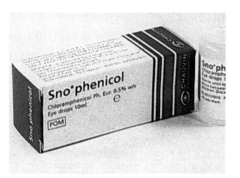

**Figure 4.12**
*Some ophthalmic products need to be refrigerated.*

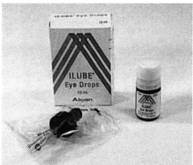

**Figure 4.13**
*EDTA can be included as a stabiliser in ophthalmic products.*

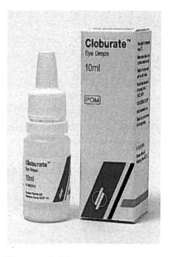

**Figure 4.14**
*Ophthalmic products containing microfine solutions.*

indicated on the packaging (Figure 4.11) where it states 'zinc sulphate 0.25% eyedrops BP'. A BP or equivalent would also be likely to indicate that the zinc sulphate eyedrops, for example, should be formulated in an aqueous solution containing boric acid.

Solutions of saline and zinc sulphate contain ingredients that are stable, but it should be noted that the manufacturers still recommend certain storage conditions and that strong light should be avoided. Therefore, while such pharmaceuticals should still be stored at 8–25°C, it is unlikely that the active ingredient will deteriorate significantly.

However, what should be noted is that even if the active ingredient could be considered as stable, the preservatives or excipients may not be. The preservative efficacy or the means to achieve solution stability could be compromised by inappropriate storage temperature, or storage beyond the expiry date. The preservative could be unstable to temperature and light (e.g. thimerosal)[21] or be absorbed into the plastic container (e.g. chlorbutanol).[22] In other cases, however, it is the active ingredient that is unstable regardless of whether pharmaceutical options exist for both brand products (e.g. POM Sno-Phenicol, Figure 4.12) or a number of generics (e.g. POM Chloramphenicol Eye Drops).

Both products of this broad-spectrum antibiotic are formulated to meet specific guidelines and should show equivalent properties. However, while chloramphenicol solutions prepared for unit-dose formulation (see Figure 4.1) are relatively stable because the drug solution is sealed into a single-use container, those in these multi-use pharmaceuticals are less stable.

Refrigeration of stocks before dispensing is essential and, once opened, the usage life is shorter than 1 month, and should be used within 21 days.

In recognising the existence of specific storage guidelines, one really needs to consider keeping the pharmaceutical refrigerated, no matter how impractical this might seem to be. Once exposed to light and air at room temperature, the antibiotic, such as chloramphenicol, can degrade to a range of reactive aldehyde and nitroso-compounds.[23] These are clinically relevant because a range of adverse effects attributed to chloramphenicol may be precipitated by these degradation products and not the parent drug.

The practical reality of these types of recommendations for limited usage life can have important clinical consequences. To use the entire contents of a 10 ml bottle of chloramphenicol would require a dosing regimen of one to two drops into the affected eye four times a day (*qds*) for 21 days. Such an extended treatment regimen for a bacterial conjunctivitis is unusual and is unlikely to be recommended nowadays for chloramphenicol.

With a reasonable starting regimen for bacterial conjunctivitis being chloramphenicol 0.5% *qds* for 7 days, and with there simply being no economic basis of marketing smaller (5 ml) bottles for such a long-used and now multigeneric product, an inevitable consequence is a partly used bottle of chloramphenicol eyedrops. Therefore, as part of initial instructions and follow-up considerations, there must be instructions on disposal of the unused portion of the pharmaceutical to reduce the risk of repeated use of a pharmaceutical that has expired and should no longer be used.

A different aspect of stability applies to ophthalmic acetylcysteine solutions (e.g. POM Ilube, Figure 4.13). Acetylcysteine is a reducing agent and, because it is able to dissociate S–S bonds in glycoproteins, it is used as a mucus-dissociating (mucolytic) agent. Ophthalmic acetylcysteine has had sporadic use over at least 30 years for severe filamentary keratitis forms of dry eye.[24] However, the extemporaneous formulation of respiratory products (by designated hospital pharmacies under the auspices of the marketing company) can result in a diluted solution that should be stored in a refrigerator at all times and used within 4–7 days. Even within this short time period, storage at room temperature can result in at least 10% loss of the active drug.[25]

However, it is possible to formulate acetylcysteine solutions with stabilisers such as EDTA which allow them to be used for much longer periods and without refrigeration.[25] This presumably applies to the product illustrated since the fine print in the ABPI lists this stabiliser as an excipient, i.e. an inactive ingredient. It is therefore essential that any patient records and literature sources pertaining to the use of an ophthalmic pharmaceutical identify the actual product used and not just the active drug.

Other therapeutic eyedrops are nominally more stable, yet are more complex and require special considerations for their use – ophthalmic corticosteroids are such an example. Clobetasone, a moderate-strength ophthalmic corticosteroid,[26]

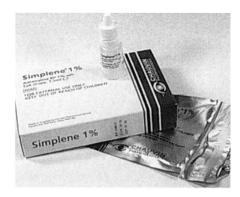

**Figure 4.15**
*Aluminium foil packaging to protect light-sensitive products.*

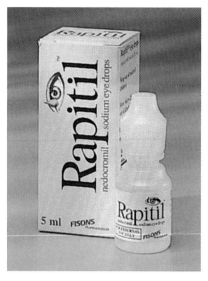

**Figure 4.16**
*Ophthalmic solutions can be coloured.*

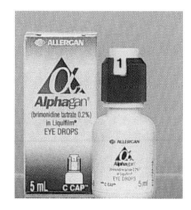

**Figure 4.17**
*C-CAP on ophthalmic pharmaceuticals for compliance.*

suitable for use in uncomplicated cases of inflammation of the conjunctiva and eyelid margins (e.g. POM Cloburate, Figure 4.14), is essentially an insoluble molecule and its persistence in solution is determined by special excipients.

In this case, it is not a true solution but a microfine suspension of the drug. If this suspension freezes, there can be reduced efficacy of the product with such a degraded product indirectly causing harm to the eye (because it did not work), or it can be rather irritating. This is an example of a product potentially compromised by extremes of temperature and a reason why ophthalmic medicines should not be left in any place at risk for such changes.

Instability to light is another important issue. Solutions of adrenaline (epinephrine) are inherently unstable because it is prone to photo-oxidation resulting in insoluble and inactive residues.[27] Ophthalmic adrenaline 1% or 2% solutions are indicated for use in the long-term management of open-angle glaucoma (see Chapter 10) and were once marketed in special amber glass bottles. With such a dark bottle, it was impossible to see how much of such an important medication was left in the bottle, and also difficult to assess whether the product had deteriorated and discoloured.

When there were a number of ophthalmic drugs susceptible to photo-oxidation, manufacture of special bottles (including dispensing of a sealed bottle with a separate sterile-packaged dropper pipette, see Figure 4.13) was generally acceptable. However, as the use and availability of such products lessened, alternative packaging methods became desirable.

Some stability can be provided by adding

antioxidants as excipients, e.g. small quantities of acetylcysteine in POM Simplene. This light-sensitive product can be made available in relatively small (7.5 ml) bottles made from clear plastic to facilitate identification of deterioration, while total protection from light during storage can be provided by an aluminium foil package (POM Simplene, Figure 4.15). Again, the BP formulation requirements can be noted on the packaging.

However, it should still be noted that the smaller bottle, used at a dosage of one drop in each eye twice daily, would still last for several weeks and could deteriorate once the light-proof foil package is opened.

As a closing note on the colour of ophthalmic solutions, it should be stressed that not all coloration is unacceptable. As noted earlier, a very slight pale amber colour to unit-dose ophthalmic chloramphenicol (see Figure 4.1) is acceptable but any substantial coloration is not; the very slight colour is all but impossible to detect for a multi-use product.

Similarly, ophthalmic solutions of pilocarpine are likely to show a very slight pale amber coloration, especially at the higher concentrations (POM Pilocarpine eye drops BP, 0.5 to 4%, see Figure 4.10) but any discoloration is also hard to detect in the multi-use bottles.

As noted earlier, some ophthalmic products deliberately include a blue colouring agent (see Figure 4.3), while other solutions have a very distinct colour, e.g.

nedocromil sodium 2% solutions (POM Rapitil, Figure 4.16). With such a distinct canary yellow colour, a slight yellowing of the tear film meniscus should be expected after use for allergic conjunctivitis.

Since past experience with colouring agents such as methylene blue shows they can slightly discolour the conjunctiva with extended use or abuse,[7] it will be interesting to learn that the same can occur with obviously coloured solutions as nedocromil sodium. As is hopefully self-evident, the use of such distinctly coloured solutions concurrent with soft contact lens wear is likely to cause discoloration of the lens matrix, so the manufacturers' guidelines, 'do not use with soft contact lenses', have to be respected. Similarly, adrenaline (epinephrine) eyedrops can substantially discolour soft contact lenses.[7]

As outlined above, most ophthalmic pharmaceuticals are now marketed in 5 ml or 10 ml white plastic bottles with white plastic caps, or in small clear plastic bottles with clear or white caps. The small bottle may be packaged in a cardboard carton or even in a foil package within a cardboard carton. There are some other variants, however.

Some medications for long-term management of open-angle glaucoma (e.g. brimonidine) are marketed in bottles that have a special screw cap that clicks into a new position each time it is opened. This is the compliance or C-CAP (e.g. POM Alphagan, Figure 4.17) designed to serve as a reminder to older patients whether they have taken both the first and second dose of the day of these important medications.

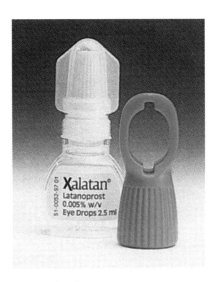

**Figure 4.18**
*Unusual types of caps for ophthalmic products.*

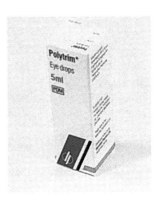

**Figure 4.19**
*Example of eyedrops containing two active ingredients.*

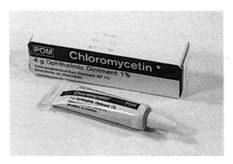

**Figure 4.21**
*Small tubes (4 g) characteristic of ophthalmic (eye) ointments.*

Another unusual type of cap can be found on products which are so small that opening them could prove difficult for elderly patients with vision or manual dexterity problems. A brightly coloured blue flanged cap-opener is provided with the very small (2.5 ml) bottle of the glaucoma drug called latanoprost, (i.e. POM Xalatan, Figure 4.18) (see Chapter 10). The very small bottle is because this drug is considered to show such efficacy in controlling IOP that it is only indicated for once-daily use, and even such a small bottle will still take nearly a month to use, at which time it should be discarded.

In terms of product options and sales, the majority of ophthalmic pharmaceuticals contain a single active ingredient. However, there have traditionally been products for general use that contain two active drugs, e.g. P Otrivine–Antistin (see Figure 4.2) contains both an alpha$_1$-adrenergic decongestant and a histamine H$_1$ blocker for use in known cases of allergic conjunctivitis.[1]

This dual pharmacological approach to management of an external eye condition does not only improve efficacy but also compliance, but it takes extra special formulation and characterisation to prepare an ophthalmic pharmaceutical containing two or more active drugs. These issues apply to allergic conjunctivitis as well as uncomplicated bacterial conjunctivitis, where two or more antibacterial drugs are included in a product to maximise the

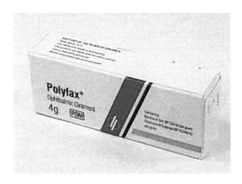

**Figure 4.20**
*Example of an eye ointment containing two active ingredients.*

chance of counteracting a bacterial infection.

For example, combinations of a sulphonamide-type antibiotic called trimethoprim and a membrane-active antibiotic called polymyxin B are available (e.g. POM Polytrim, Figure 4.19). Such products should provide coverage against a wide spectrum of organisms that can be expected to precipitate bacterial conjunctivitis (see Chapter 8) and are for use on a *qds* basis (again with a nominal regimen for 7 days, or for 1–2 days after the apparent infection has resolved).

Similar combinations can be found for ophthalmic antibiotic ointments for use in blepharoconjunctivitis,[7] including recurrent cases, where a membrane-active antibiotic such as polymyxin B is now combined with a specific antibiotic active on the cell walls of Gram-positive bacteria, bacitracin zinc (e.g. POM Polyfax Ophthalmic Ointment, Figure 4.20). Such a product can be used just twice daily but

should be applied carefully to the eyelid margins to ensure maximum efficacy.

In the case of antibiotic mixtures, the BP designation is important not only for the ophthalmic formulation but also the special purity of the antibiotic. For example, the '10,000 U/gram' designation for the polymyxin B stipulates the expected antibacterial efficacy of that drug quantity where the U stands for an internationally accepted unit of activity.

Another point that should be noted about ophthalmic ointments is that the dispensed quantity is small, e.g. 4 g (Figure 4.20). The same also applies for eye ointments containing a single antibiotic such as chloramphenicol (e.g. POM Chloromycetin, Figure 4.21) or a single corticosteroid (e.g. POM Hydrocortisone Eye Ointment, Figure 4.22). Such smaller tube sizes are typical and very different from similar products that are designated for topical skin use (e.g. POM Polyfax available as a 20 g tube), or the numerous topical skin products containing 1% hydrocortisone available in 20–30 g tubes.

The topical skin products are not for ophthalmic use under any circumstances. The largest and somewhat oversized ophthalmic gel products currently available are 10 g, introduced originally as hospital products (e.g. P Gel Tears), but now also available in 5 g tubes.

As with eyedrops, these small tubes of ophthalmic antibiotics, corticosteroids or even unmedicated (bland) ointments are also designed to be compatible with both the expected use and to minimise complications. It has long been recommended (e.g. *BPC* (1973)), but not always accepted that, once opened, all ophthalmic ointments should be discarded after one month. Some products will carry this specific instruction on the carton.

The formulation of chloramphenicol in an ointment base and in a lightproof tube means the drug is more stable than in eyedrops. Some consideration of its storage is still necessary and the company recommends storage at temperatures less than 30°C.

An antibiotic ophthalmic ointment contains a drug dispersed in a mixture of a petrolatum base with wool fat, with or without lanolin. The specifics of the ingredients and their purity is very important.[14,28,29] Regardless, the resultant material is 'greasy' and has limited miscibility with the tear film. It usually has to be stable at room temperature for storage.

The ophthalmic ointment is designed to prolong the contact of the medication with the surface of the eye rather than it being rapidly washed away (Chapter 2). There are two aspects to ointments that can receive adverse press, both of which can readily be countered. These aspects relate to vision and compatibility.

First, it is often stated that ophthalmic ointments are messy and degrade vision and so perhaps should even be avoided or only used under an eye patch. However, some of these problems surely only arise because a patient has been left to decide how much ointment to apply and exactly how to apply it. It takes but a few moments to demonstrate that a 1 cm (half-inch) ribbon is all that is needed for each dose and that it can be carefully extruded into the lower cul-de-sac.

For recurrent lid conditions, judicious application of even smaller amounts along the eye lid margins may be all that is needed, so a patient does not necessarily have to endure 'blurry vision' for 10–15 minutes after application of the ointment (although the patient should be advised that such vision decrease could be suffered for a couple of minutes).

A compatibility issue relates to vision after the use of ointments and the potential – in rare cases – of an allergic reaction to the ointment ingredients. A key ingredient here is lanolin, which not only has known allergenic potential but, is in reality, provided with every opportunity to elicit a reaction simply because the formulation is designed for prolonged contact.

There does not seem to be a consistency to reporting on the lanolin content of currently marketed ophthalmic ointments so

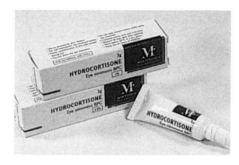

**Figure 4.22**
*Small tubes (3 g) characteristic of ophthalmic (eye) corticosteroid ointments.*

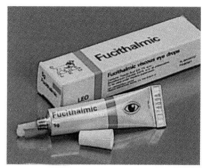

**Figure 4.23**
*Ophthalmic gels.*

the point should be made that the persistence of oedematous and irritated eyelids during therapy could be caused by the treatment (and should resolve promptly when the offending product is discontinued and an appropriate alternative substituted). Such reaction of the eyelid margins or conjunctival chemosis can be both a cause of substantial patient discomfort and is cosmetically unappealing.

Where this happens, judicious application over a period of 3–5 days of other ophthalmic ointments containing anti-inflammatory drugs can be of great benefit (e.g. POM Hydrocortisone Eye Ointment 1% or 2.5%, see Figure 4.22).

As with antibiotic ointments, a little patient education on how to apply the required dose of such anti-inflammatory products, especially to the eyelid margins, can make a major difference to their efficacy and reduce the chance of adverse reactions developing simply because there is no inadvertent overdosing.

The use of ophthalmic ointments can provide a most useful option in primary eye care in that compliance with therapies for bacterial blepharoconjunctivitis or severe dry-eye conditions can be better when an ointment is used. As noted above, the adverse press on ointments can sometime negate this advance. However, there is a modern-day alternative in the form of the ophthalmic gel.

These largely transparent gels have a consistency that is not dissimilar to ophthalmic ointments yet they do not have the greasy characteristics of traditional eye ointments. These gels are actually very viscous solutions of polymers of acrylic acid known under the proprietary name of Carbomer (e.g. Carbomer 934 in POM Fucithalmic, Figure 4.23). The vehicle for the

antibiotic in this case is now the Carbomer gel, which should provide equivalent extended contact at the ocular surface to an ointment formulation.

More importantly, just as twice-daily (*bds*) use of a chloramphenicol ophthalmic ointment for conjunctivitis can be as effective as *qds* eyedrops containing the same antibiotic, the ophthalmic gel (e.g. of fusidic acid) can provide this *bds* dosing option with much less chance of significant messiness and blurring of vision.[30]

In their early use some 10 years ago, some ophthalmic gels received adverse press because a mild 'toxic' keratitis could develop with extended use over many weeks to months. It should be noted, however, that the effect could be due either to the gel or the simple fact that drugs in the gel now have prolonged contact with the corneal surface. While this matter remains to be resolved, it appears unlikely that ophthalmic antibiotic gels or those marketed as ophthalmic lubricants (e.g. P Viscotears or P GelTears) will precipitate such an adverse effect.

## General characteristics of the pharmaceutical vehicle

The vehicle for a drug is the basis for classification of ophthalmic pharmaceutical types, and is the proper term to describe the delivery system in which the drug is dissolved or dispersed.

Aqueous solutions are those products formulated for use as eyedrops or as irrigating solutions and can be expected to have an osmolality and pH similar to tears. In some cases, a drug is not readily soluble so suspensions are made which should be gently shaken just before use if the desired clinical effect is to be achieved.

The stability of an ophthalmic pharmaceutical is determined primarily by the pH of the solution. This pH is that at which the drug(s) show the slowest rate of chemical breakdown, and it is important that the pH-adjusting chemicals are stable. Simple solutions of NaCl (saline) containing phosphate buffers or borate buffers are very stable, but solutions containing carbonate or tromethamine are less stable.

The stability is also influenced by the osmolality of a solution, which can only be maintained if the bottle cap is kept on. The actual concentration of the active ingredient(s) in a pharmaceutical are also important in determining that the specified drug concentration is within certain limits and stays that way. This requirement implies that the active ingredient is stable in its vehicle, and with all the other ingredients and additives (e.g. stabilisers, preservatives and polymers). If commercial products are diluted, they may then be unstable.

To ensure that these stability requirements are realised, a pharmaceutical has a specified shelf life (i.e. the time period between the manufacture and the expiration date). The stability may also be maintained through the use of 'stabilisers'. The various stabilisers most commonly included in these pharmaceuticals serve as anti-oxidants, e.g. sodium metabisulphite (often referred to as bisulphites), low concentrations of N-acetylcysteine or EDTA (usually called disodium edetate, or edetate sodium). Such reducing agents will reduce the oxygen-dependent degradation of the active ingredient (e.g. topical ocular anaesthetics, or adrenaline eyedrops).

Last but not least, a reasonable means of maintaining sterility is really required for any product designated for multiple use. This is achieved with preservatives.[14,29] Several different preservatives are used but benzalkonium chloride is most commonly used in the UK at this time. This quaternary ammonium compound is a cationic compound with surface-active (surfactant) properties and is nowadays included at concentrations of just 0.004%, much less than the concentration (0.02%) where a toxic keratitis or conjunctivitis would likely develop. Cetrimide (also known as cetrimonium or cetyltrimethylammonium bromide) is another quaternary ammonium cationic surfactant used at the 0.005 to 0.01% concentration.

Other preservatives include benzethonium chloride, polidronium (Polyquad), benzododecinium bromide, polixetonium (a water-soluble – Cationic Polymer, WSCP), chlorbutol (also known as chlor(o)butanol), chlorhexidine, thimerosal, p-hydroxybenzoate, phenylethyl alcohol, myristyl-gamma-picolinium chloride, parabens, methyl-parabens, propyl-parabens and phenylmercuric nitrate or acetate.

Assuming that all the above considerations and precautions relating to ophthalmic preparations are respected, it is still necessary to inspect each and every pharmaceutical before use, whether it be unit-dose or multidose. Degraded solutions may show a slight or substantial colour change (e.g. yellow or even orange brown in rare cases for ophthalmic anaesthetic solutions) or contain fine to coarse precipitates. These degradation products may only be evident as a slight discoloration around the dropper tip.

In summary, ophthalmic products represent a special category of pharmaceuticals formulated to meet special requirements in terms of drug delivery and safety. Knowledge of the formulation requirements and the characteristics of the products is an essential part of the selection of these pharmaceuticals in primary eye care, with different pharmaceuticals being indicated not only for various conditions but also with different dosing regimens.

# References

1 Doughty MJ (1997) A guide to ophthalmic pharmacy medicines in the United Kingdom. *Ophthal Physiol Opt* **17** (suppl 1): S2–S8.

2 Anon (1997) OOs to supply hayfever drug. *Optician* **213**: 4.

3 Anon (1997) Mail order regulation. *Pharmaceut J* **258**: 753.

4 German EJ, Hurst MA, Wood D (1997) Eye drop container delivery: a source of response variation? *Ophthal Physiol Opt* **17**: 196–204.

5 Medicine, Ethics and Practice, No. 22 (1999, July) Royal Pharmaceutical Society of Great Britain.

6 Robert G (1920) Note sur l'emploi du blue de méthylène en thérapeutique oculaire. *Ann d'Oculist* **157**: 507–509.

7 Doughty MJ (1996) Diagnostic and therapeutic pharmaceutical agents for use in contact lens practice. In: *Clinical Contact Lens Practice* (Bennett ED, Weissman BA, eds). JB Lippincott, Philadelphia, USA Chapter 9, pp. 1–38.

8 Doughty MJ (1994) Acute effects of chlorobutanol- or benzalkonium chloride-containing artificial tears on the surface features of rabbit corneal epithelial cells. *Optom Vis Sci* **7**: 562–571.

9 Rubinstein MP, Evans JE (1997) Therapeutic contact lenses and eye-drops – is there a problem? *Contact Lens Anterior Eye* **20**: 9–11.

10 Doughty MJ (1999) Re-wetting, comfort, lubricant and moisturising solutions for the contact lens wearer. *Contact Lens Anterior Eye* **22**: 116–126.

11 Christensen MT, Bary JR, Turner FD (1998) Five-minute removal of soft lenses prevents most absorption of a topical ophthalmic solution. *CLAO J* **24**: 227–231.

12 Doughty MJ (1996) Sodium cromoglycate ophthalmic solution as a pharmacy medicine for the management of mild-to-moderate, non-infectious inflammation of the conjunctiva in adults. *Ophthal Physiol Opt* **16** (suppl 2): S33–S38.

13 Wood CA (1909) *A System of Ophthalmic Therapeutics*. Cleveland Press, Chicago.

14 Doughty MJ (1991) Basic principles of pharmacology. In: *Clinical Ocular Pharmacology and Therapeutics* (Onofrey B, ed). JB Lippincott, Philadelphia, USA Chapter 1, pp. 1–38.

15 Pearson FC (1990) *Aseptic Pharmaceutical Manufacturing Technology for the 1990s* (Olson WP, Groves MJ, eds), pp. 75–100.

16 O'Connor Davies PH (1972) *The Actions and Uses of Ophthalmic Drugs*. Barrie & Jenkins, London, UK.

17 Fletcher EL, Brennan NA (1993) The effect of solution tonicity on the eye. *Clin Exptl Optom* **76**: 17–21.

18 Trolle-Lassen C (1958) Investigations into the sensitivity of the human eye to hypo- and hypertonic solutions as well as solutions with unphysiological hydrogen ion concentrations. *Pharm Weekbl Sci* **93**: 148–153.

19 Conrad JM, Reay WA, Polcyn RE *et al.* (1978) Influence of tonicity and pH on lacrimation and ocular drug bioavailability. *J Parenter Drug Assoc* **32**: 149–161.

20 Norn M (1985) Tear pH after instillation of buffer in vivo. *Acta Ophthalmol* **63** (S.173): 32–34.

21 Caraballo I, Rabasco AM, Fernandez Revalo M (1993) Study of thimerosal degradation mechanism. *Int J Pharmaceut* **89**: 213–221.

22 Dunn DL, Jones WJ, Dorsey ED (1983) Analysis of chlorobutanol in ophthalmic ointments and aqueous solutions by reverse phase high-performance liquid chromatography. *J Pharm Sci* **72**: 277–280.

23 de Vries H, Van Henegouwen GMJB, Huf FA (1984) Photochemical decomposition of chloramphenicol in a 0.25 percent eyedrop and in a therapeutic intraocular concentration. *Int J Pharmaceut* **20**: 265–271.

24 Doughty MJ (1990) What is really new and where do we go from here for dry and irritated eyes? *Optom Vis Sci* **67**: 567–571.

25 Anaizi NH, Swenson CF, Dentinger PJ (1997) Stability of acetylcysteine in an extempraneously compounded ophthalmic solution. *Am J Health-Syst Pharm* **54**: 549–552.

26 Kadom AH, Forrester JV, Williamson TH (1986) Comparison of the anti-inflammatory activity and effect on intraocular pressure of flouromethalone, clobetasone butyrate and betamethasone phosphate eye drops. *Ophthal Physiol Opt* **6**: 313–17.

27 McCarthy RW, LeBlanc R (1976) A 'black cornea' secondary to topical epinephrine. *Can J Ophthalmol* **11**: 336–340.

28 De Muynck C, Lalljie SP, Sandra P et al. (1993) Chemical and physicochemical characterization of petrolatums used in eye ointment formulations. *J Pharm Pharmacol* **45**: 500–503.

29 Mullen W, Shepherd W, Labovitz J (1973) Ophthalmic preservatives and vehicles. *Surv Ophthalmol* **17**: 469–483.

30 Sinclair NM, Leigh DA (1988) A comparison of fusidic acid and viscous eye drops and chloramphenicol eye ointment in acute conjunctivitis. *Curr Therap Res Clin Exptl* **44**: 468–474.

# 5
# Medication-related adverse drug reactions (ADRs) and the anterior eye tissues

Medication-related adverse drug reactions and the anterior eye
General perspectives on detection and monitoring
Systemic medications and the eyelid skin
Systemic medications and the conjunctiva
Systemic medications and tears
Systemic medications and the cornea
Systemic medications and the anterior crystalline lens

## Introduction

An established role of optometrists is to detect any ocular abnormality and, under current regulations, generally refer such patients to a GP or to the hospital service.[1] With a role of optometric provision of primary eye care, it is logical that a range of these abnormalities should no longer be considered as necessary referrals but that high-street optometrists would assume responsibility for full evaluation of patients and their management.[1,2]

One particular area of ocular 'abnormalities' is that associated with the use of systemic medications by patients. In this module, the types of systemic medication-related (iatrogenic) alterations in the tissues and cells of the anterior eye will be considered.

Decisions on the health of the external eye need to take into account whether a patient's medications could be a cause of an abnormality, or influence the course of any natural condition or disease. Certain medication groups need to be considered and management options adjusted accordingly. Overall, however, the recognition of these iatrogenic changes is an essential part of

the management of anterior eye disease. The use of systemic medications could exacerbate a disease process (e.g. dry eye), interfere with the recognition of a true disease or otherwise detract attention from a disease process.

In this chapter, the types of systemic medication-related (iatrogenic) alterations to the tissues and cells of the anterior eye will be considered. For the anterior eye (eyelids, lacrimal system, conjunctiva, cornea and anterior crystalline lens) it is unlikely that these iatrogenic changes will result in major complications, so an optometrist's role should be to undertake a series of tests, provide appropriate counsel to patients and consider whether the eye is at risk for any specific problem that could require further specific management. For example, where a function such as lacrimation is affected, the management of the patient should logically go beyond detection and monitoring, but include the provision of palliative care.

When systemic medications affect the tissues of the anterior eye, it is unlikely that just one of these tissues will be affected. While the effects on one tissue may be more pronounced, the very fact

that changes have occurred, or could occur, requires that the clinical assessment consider all these components.

Many of the iatrogenic changes that will be considered in this module are reported retrospectively and the published case reports or retrospective reporting systems (e.g. the yellow card scheme (Figure 5.1)) rarely contain a full set of clinical details. However, an attempt will be made to consider how all these components of the anterior eye can be affected by systemic medications (Table 5.1).

## General perspectives on detection and monitoring

From a perspective of which adverse drug reactions (ADRs) might most commonly be encountered, it is the lacrimal system that is likely to be the most sensitive to a range of systemic medications, including those active on the sympathetic and parasympathetic systems of the body.

Any change in the lacrimal system will affect the tear film and can, in the extreme, produce changes in the conjunctiva and cornea resembling dry-eye type diseases.

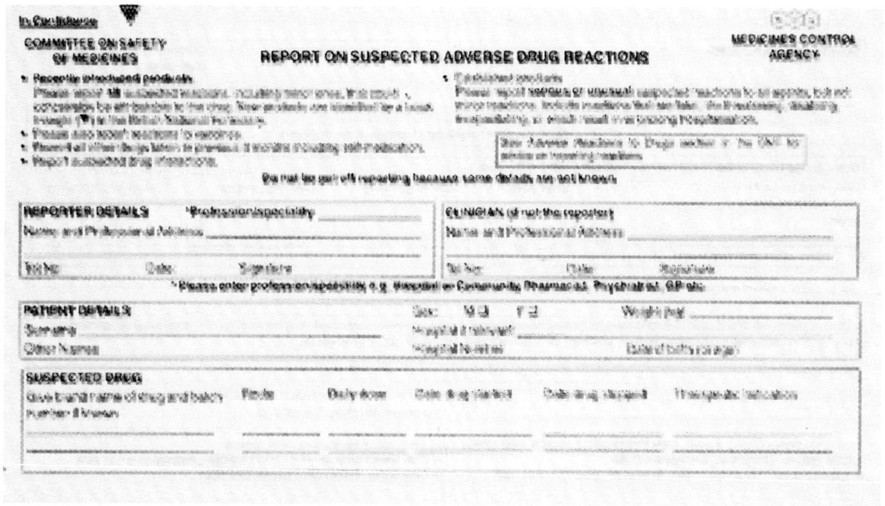

**Figure 5.1**
*A sample 'yellow card'.*

Other drugs can exert effects directly on the health of the conjunctiva and indirectly affect the tear film. Some of these drugs, as well as others, can cause a unique photosensitivity that results in drug deposits developing in the conjunctiva, cornea or lens, yet may not obviously have effects on the tear film. Such photosensitivity may also extend to the external eyelid skin and provide an indication that a patient could be at risk of ocular changes.

A systems approach can be adopted in that each component of the anterior eye should be evaluated systematically and appropriate notes made on a patient's records (Figure 5.2). Most of these iatrogenic events are noted in pharmaceutical directories such as *MIMS* or the *BNF*, although it is uncommon for specific terms relating to the eye to be used. Further details can be found in an *ABPI Data Sheet Compendium* (see Chapter 1).

Any time that patients' medical histories indicate that they are on medications which could affect the appearance of the anterior eye, their records should clearly indicate that specific checks were done, for instance by making statements to show that each part of the eye was evaluated. Some of these notes can be in an accepted abbreviated form, e.g. 'cornea – biomicroscopy WNL' would indicate that there was nothing remarkable ('within normal limits') about the appearance of the cornea and that there was no obvious oedema, no obvious adherent material, deposits or

opacities, but does unambiguously record that an evaluation was done.

Evaluation of the bulbar conjunctiva or palpebral conjunctiva similarly can be performed by biomicroscopy or even the naked eye and appropriate notes or grading schemes used similar to those employed for contact lens wear-related complications,[3] e.g. 'grade 1 = trace intra-epithelial deposits – no clinical action required'.

A sketch of where the deposits were located is an important part of any patient's record (Figure 5.2). Again, such notes not only indicate that an evaluation was done but that its relative magnitude was also assessed.

While no clinical action was required, these assessments are essential if the recovery and/or progression of the iatrogenic events are to be achieved effectively. In other cases, however, it must be accepted that visual examination *per se* is not sufficient, so the notes in patients' records should also indicate that the evaluation was carried out with appropriate diagnostic drugs.

For example, if the condition of the corneal surface is to be assessed, then fluorescein dye must be used and the records could then indicate 'corneal surface with fluorescein – WNL'. This indicates that while the patient had no iatrogenic condition affecting his or her corneal epithelium, an evaluation with sufficient sensitivity was performed to rule out subtle

changes not readily detectable by unaided biomicroscopy.

Similarly, the technique and circumstance under which the crystalline lens was examined is essential, and in the opinion of this writer, should always be done before and after pupil dilation so that both the potential impact of any cataractous change on vision can be guessed at

**Table 5.1  Systemic medications and the external and anterior eye tissues**

Decisions on the health of the anterior eye need to take into account whether a patient's medications could be a cause of an abnormality or influence the course of any natural condition or disease.

*Eyelid skin pigmentary changes*
  tetracyclines
  phenothiazines
  amiodarone
  gold salts

*Conjunctival pigmentary changes*
  tetracyclines
  phenothiazines

*Conjunctival irritation/hyperaemia*
  isotretinoin
  anti-cancer drugs
  HRT (conjugated oestrogens)
  alpha-adrenergic blockers

*Lacrimal hyposecretion*
  thiazide diuretics
  oral $H_1$ blocking antihistamines
  benzodiazepines
  tricyclic antidepressants
  tetracyclic antidepressants
  oral beta-adrenergic blockers

*Corneal deposits*
  phenothiazines
  gold salts
  amiodarone
  flecainide
  chloroquine
  hydroxychloroquine
  tamoxifen

*Corneal surface changes (SPK)*
  phenothiazines?
  anti-cancer drugs
  NSAIDs

*Anterior lens deposits*
  phenothiazines
  amiodarone
  benzodiazepines

ANTERIOR EYE TISSUES

|  | Right | Left |
|---|---|---|
| General appearance | | |
| Eyelid skin and margins | | |
| Bulbar conjunctiva | | |
| Palpebral conjunctiva | | |
| Limbus | | |
| Cornea | | |
| Tear break-up time | | |
| Other tests | | |
| Anterior chamber | | |
| Anterior chamber angle | | |
| Iris | | |
| Pupil size | | |

Lens
IOP _____  Time

Techniques

☐ Slit lamp ☐ Binocular indirect ☐ Tonometry

Pharmaceuticals use

| Time | Pharmaceutical | Dose | Eye(s) |
|---|---|---|---|
| | | | |

**Figure 5.2**
*Each component of the anterior eye should be systematically evaluated and appropriate notes made on a patient's records.*

(with the normal pupil) and the true extent of any changes seen (following dilation).

The records thus must show a pupil dilation was performed, the pharmaceuticals used and when. Obviously, if the drug(s) causing the cataractous changes can also affect the pupil then the records should clearly indicate that this was considered.

In other cases, clinical experience indicates that some form of specific test really should be done to obtain a measure of the functional integrity of the tear film by a tear break-up time measure,[4] or perhaps a Schirmer test.[5] Whether or not the patient is also symptomatic is also now very important since such information should guide the management of the condition. As with other details, these symptoms should be noted on patients' records so that any therapies can be systematically adjusted in response to these patients' needs.

Last, and not least, any considerations of changes in cosmetic appearance of the eyelids or bulbar conjunctiva should be done within the context of a patient's use

of cosmetics; that questions have been asked in this area and the appropriate details should also be noted in patients' records.

## Systemic medications and the eyelid skin

The surface of the eyelids will often be exposed to the sun and so, just as with the forehead and facial skin, is prone to light sensitivity. A limited range of systemic drugs can act as photosensitisers in that concurrent sunlight exposure can result in a photo-induced ADR.

In the extreme, such photosensitisation can lead to a progressive and marked 'tanning' of the skin but this does not necessarily develop uniformly. As a result, and obviously depending upon patients' natural skin tones, the skin can develop brown, slate grey or purplish discoloration or variant shades in between. These can be localised to discrete regions on the eyelids or periocular skin (Figure 5.3).

The discoloration is the result of pigment accumulation resulting from photodegradation of drugs, so the degree of discoloration is probably related to lifestyle (i.e. exposure to the sun and an out-of-doors occupation or leisure lifestyle). However, the possibility of drug-induced purpura should not be overlooked.

Such changes can occur with chronic use of drugs including tetracycline antibiotics such as minocycline,[6] phenothiazine neuroleptic drugs such as chlorpromazine,[7] amiodarone for severe cardiac arrhythmias,[8] or gold salts for refractory rheumatoid arthritis.[9] Oral isotretinoin therapy for severe acne can also produce erythematous photosensitivity. It is unlikely to show

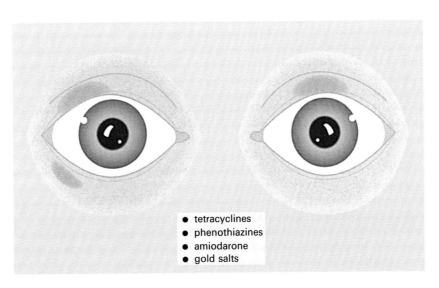

- tetracyclines
- phenothiazines
- amiodarone
- gold salts

**Figure 5.3**
*Eyelid skin pigmentary changes showing hyperpigmentation of eyelid skin.*

distinct coloration,[10] but may be especially noticeable because of concurrent conjunctival changes (see below).

While there may be some discomfort (e.g. a general urticaria with tetracyclines), the management generally requires limiting sunlight exposure since it is often not a simple matter of discontinuing the offending medications and substituting something else.

## Systemic medications and the conjunctiva

A number of systemic medications can produce a conjunctivitis or blepharoconjunctivitis and it is very important that different types of effects are distinguished from each other and from a range of eyelid margin and conjunctival diseases.

The first type of reactions produce cosmetic changes that are the result of photosensitisation. The conjunctiva, especially within the palpebral aperture, is also generally exposed to the sunlight and photosensitivity reactions may well develop concurrently with eyelid skin changes. Normal spectacle lenses appear unlikely to protect the conjunctiva and cornea from such changes.

Deposits or generalised pigmentary changes can develop in the conjunctival epithelia and may be largely uniform, discretely localised or clumped, but generally can be expected to be within the normal palpebral aperture (Figure 5.4).

They can have a range of colours according to the drug type and the extent of the manifest change will depend on the normal colour, vasculature and pigment in a patient's conjunctiva. Examples include chronic use of tetracycline antibiotics,[11] or chronic use of phenothiazine drugs.[12]

In most cases, these changes have little consequence other than that they are unwelcome cosmetic changes. In more severe cases, however, and probably when there is some concurrent underlying inflammation of the conjunctiva, cysts with pigmentary deposits can develop and are then generally associated with some irritation and discomfort. Overall, the location and extent of such changes should be noted in patient files but there is little else to be done. Certainly, these types of changes are not a reason for altering the medications, although a different lifestyle, limiting sunlight exposure, may be appropriate, as

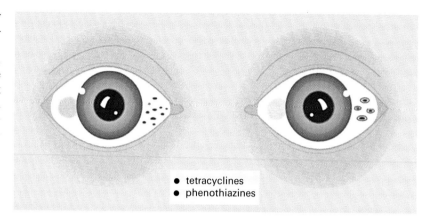

● tetracyclines
● phenothiazines

**Figure 5.4**
*Conjunctival pigmentary changes showing discoloration, patchy pigmentation (left) or pigmented cysts (right) on the bulbar conjunctiva.*

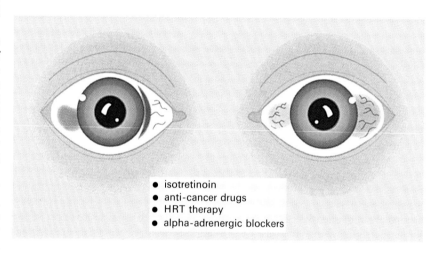

● isotretinoin
● anti-cancer drugs
● HRT therapy
● alpha-adrenergic blockers

**Figure 5.5**
*Conjunctival irritation/hyperaemia.*

with eyelid changes. Cystic inclusions might, however, need treatment.

However, another group of systemic medications can result in substantial conjunctival discomfort (Figure 5.5). Such changes are associated invariably with tear film deficiencies and lead to a 'rough' conjunctiva where there is little or no surface light reflex, concurrent with some degree of redness and irritation as well. There is likely to be concurrent irritation of eyelid margin, and especially the meibomian glands.

Evidence suggests that certain drugs directly or indirectly affect the mucus layer of the ocular surface. The general redness of the eye and the degree of patient discomfort are both important to note. Any dose of oral isotretinoin for severe acne is likely

to produce an irritating conjunctivitis,[10,13] since the drug apparently reduces mucous secretion from the goblet cells of the bulbar and palpebral conjunctiva.

It should be noted that since the period of therapy is usually for a fixed period (e.g. 8 or 12 weeks), the condition should resolve when the therapy is ended.[13] A slightly different type of irritative conjunctivitis is expected from the use of a range of oral anti-cancer drugs (e.g. cytarabine or cyclophosphamide)[14,15] because the mucous epithelia of the ocular surface, as with other similar surfaces in the body, are very susceptible to the cytotoxic effects of these drugs.

Medication groups may become notorious for their potential to produce irritative conjunctivitis, but it is important that the current drugs and their relative doses are considered before jumping to conclusions. Two notable examples are worthy of mention here.

In the 1960s, the early use of high-dose birth-control pills resulted in many anecdotal reports of conjunctivitis or even substantial tear film or corneal changes.[16–19] While any woman regularly receiving such therapy may undergo cyclical changes on ocular discomfort (in part associated with hormonal cycles) that may well limit her tolerance to contact lens wear, the potential for such changes is much less with modern-day, low-dose formulations.[17] Notwithstanding, borderline dry-eye symptoms may still be reported.[19]

Attention to older women receiving hormone replacement therapy (HRT) for menopause is probably more appropriate nowadays,[18] with the combined influences of an ageing lacrimal and glandular system along with the oestrogenic therapy likely being synergistic. It can be noted, however, that while clinically significant signs and symptoms are less likely nowadays, there is good evidence that even modern birth-control pills can produce changes in conjunctival circulation.[20]

A second notable example here is the systemic use of beta-adrenergic blockers, especially those that are selective for beta$_1$ (cardiac) receptors, e.g. atenolol. These are widely used for high blood pressure, angina and even migraine prophylaxis, yet most can be expected to produce no more than mild lacrimal hyposecretion concurrent with irritated eyes.[21]

However, one particular drug called practolol precipitated a most unusual rash associated with granulomatous conjunctivitis,[22] or simply severe dry eye.[23] From a clinical perspective, this oculomucocutaneous syndrome appears to be unique to practolol and although the true reasons for it do not appear to have been fully established, it had two consequences. First, the drug was withdrawn. Secondly, the UK pharmaceutical directories (e.g. *MIMS*) still carry a small note that systemic beta-blocker therapy should be gradually withdrawn if a severe dry eye-type condition develops. Similarly, patient information leaflets even for beta$_1$-selective beta-blockers, state that dry eyes is a possible adverse reaction.

Alpha$_1$-adrenergic blockers (e.g. prazosin, used to manage high blood

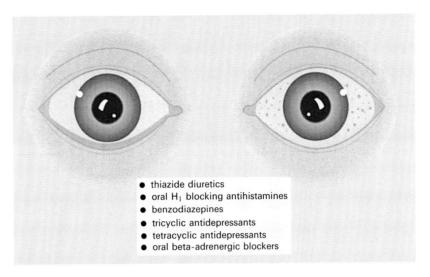

- thiazide diuretics
- oral H$_1$ blocking antihistamines
- benzodiazepines
- tricyclic antidepressants
- tetracyclic antidepressants
- oral beta-adrenergic blockers

**Figure 5.6**
*Lacrimal hyposecretion leading to dry eye with diffuse fluorescein staining.*

pressure) or drugs with these actions in addition to others (e.g. sertindole, used for schizophrenia, and carvedilol, used for high blood pressure) can cause a general peripheral vasodilation and so have occasionally been reported to cause conjunctival as well as nasal congestion; it is the latter side-effect that is more commonly listed.

Management of irritative conjunctivitis associated with isotretinoin, anti-cancer drugs, birth-control pills or HRT, generally requires counselling and the adjunct use of artificial tears (e.g. P Liquifilm Tears or equivalent).[24] Preservative-free products are unlikely to be needed; neither are true lubricants.

## Systemic medications and tears

A certain quantity of lacrimal secretion is required to maintain a normal tear film. The balance between secretion, evaporation and tear film drainage will be different for each patient so the effects are relative only.

From a practical perspective, lacrimal hyposecretion is that which is lower than that required to maintain a stable tear film volume and can lead to irritation and foreign body sensation, increased susceptibility to irritants, reduced or poor tolerance to contact lenses or poor prognosis for successful use. Evaluation and monitoring should include biomicroscopy (of tear film meniscus), tear film stability and Schirmer

test. A patient diary can help identify whether the borderline dry eye-type condition is indeed associated with medication use.

A number of drugs are frequently implicated.[19,25–27] (Figure 5.6). These drugs probably directly reduce lacrimal secretion *per se* although the mechanisms have yet to be really defined. It is important to note that these iatrogenic reductions in lacrimal secretion are likely to be time dependent in relation to when the medications were taken and also be proportional to the dose of the medication. Dry eyes *per se* are rarely mentioned in ADR lists but rather conditions such as dry mouth, or thirst.

Notwithstanding, the result is that a patient may simply periodically experience an hour or two of borderline dry-eye symptoms. Slight reductions in lacrimal secretion (Schirmer test) can be measured following the use of (higher doses of) oral diuretics such as the thiazide diuretics (e.g. hydrochlorothiazide),[28] or oral H$_1$ blocking antihistamines of the sedating type (e.g. chlorpheniramine).[29] Sedating antihistamines (e.g. promazine) can also be used for control of nausea, etc.

Similar effects would be expected following the use of any peripherally acting atropine-like (parasympatholytic) drug (e.g. oral hyoscine, oral propantheline, oral dicyclomine, skin patches containing hyoscine, etc, as used for gastrointestinal upset and travel sickness) or any other drug that has such peripheral cholinergic blocking (anticholinergic) actions as an

ADR (e.g. tricyclic antidepressants such as trimipramine, used as sleep aids).

Other drugs that can also cause similar effects include the benzodiazepine neuroleptics (e.g. oral nitrazepam, used as a sleep aid), other benzodiazepines used as anxiolytics (e.g. oral diazepam), the select dopaminergic blockers used as anxiolytics (e.g. buspirone), or other non-specific dopaminergic blockers such as the phenothiazines (e.g. chlorpromazine).

These effects can be attributed partly to true lacrimal hyposecretion with drug actions on the glands and a combined effect with the various antihistamines and anxiolytics, of a disturbance in the normal lid–tear film interactions, including spontaneous eyeblink characteristics. Anticholinergic or CNS disturbances are the ADR categories that should be looked for in *MIMS* or an equivalent directory rather than their being an explicit statement about dry eyes. It is only in extreme cases that the use of atropine-like drugs, concurrent with high bioavailability, will result in really substantial effects on the lacrimal system,[30] but even here these effects may be less noticed by a patient because of more dominant effects on the pupil or accommodation (see Chapter 7). Systemic beta-adrenergic blocking drugs (e.g. propranolol) generally can be expected adversely to affect lacrimal secretion and/or the quality of the tears.[21,31]

It is uncertain at this time whether alpha$_1$-adrenergic blocking drugs (e.g. prazosin) will change lacrimal secretion. However, various anecdotal reports have indicated that use of CNS-acting alpha$_2$-adrenergics (e.g. oral clonidine) could reduce lacrimal secretion as well as cause hyperaemia and so 'conjunctivitis' can be listed as an ADR. However, such alpha$_2$ regulation of tear flow is unproven.[32]

For diuretics or beta-adrenergic antagonists (or even alpha$_2$-agonists), while the dose can be adjusted or a different combination used, the patient needs these medications for a medical condition that is far more serious than dry eye. For oral antihistamines, the 'drying' effect is often a wanted property of these drugs to manage the nasal and upper respiratory tract symptoms and so, as with the use of diuretics, it is an ADR that has to be managed rather than the drug being discontinued.

Once a patient needs routine use of sleep aids, antidepressants or anxiolytics, any

lacrimal deficiencies generally require symptomatic management rather than considering discontinuation. Overall therefore, medication-related lacrimal deficiency should be managed with a fixed regimen of artificial tears. As with conjunctival irritation, preservative-containing, multidose 'artificial tear' products should be adequate in the majority of patients.

Various anecdotal reports indicate that excessive consumption of ethyl alcohol or caffeine can be problematic. Some practitioners have noted anecdotally that a reduction in their intake can both increase ocular comfort and improve contact lens intolerance. These drugs therefore presumably cause lacrimal hyposecretion and also disturbance in tear film – eye blink interaction.

The opposite effect is uncommon but should not be ignored for lacrimal hypersecretion may produce a 'dishwasher hands' type of cornea and conjunctiva and can require judicious use of lubricants or lubricating ointments (a wet dry eye). A lacrimal hypersecretion can be considered as any level of tear production that is higher than that required to maintain a fully-wetted ocular surface and normal tear film thickness, and can also be expected to be associated with tear film instability. It may be the indirect result of suboptimal lacrimal drainage and may also be accompanied by lid margin oedema.

Allergies can produce similar hypersecretion and excessive use of topical nasal decongestants (e.g. those containing xylometazoline) could produce a 'rebound effect' that causes hypersecretion.[24,27]

On a more serious note, there is the potential for narcotic opioid analgesics (e.g. oral morphine, etc) or indirect-acting cholinergics (anticholinesterases) as medications for muscular dystonia (e.g. oral neostigmine) to cause lacrimal hypersecretion and a patient may only report unwanted moist eyes, yet will wet the entire length of a Schirmer strip when tested. It will be interesting to see whether newly-marketed anticholinesterases such as donepezil will produce any ocular symptoms in the older group of patients most likely to be on this medication (for Alzheimer's disease).

The lacrimal hypersecretory effect can be used to advantage and low doses of direct-acting cholinergics (e.g. oral pilocarpine, POM Salagen) could promote lacrimal secretion in patients with severe dry eyes.

In the UK, these drugs are indicated for promoting salivary secretion in patients with Sjögren's syndrome rather than being specifically indicated for a lacrimal effect.

Lastly, it should be noted that some drugs, such as those for cancer, can produce a general toxic reaction to the conjunctival membranes (e.g. oral cytarabine, cyclophosphamide) and as a result of the chronic irritation, hypersecretion and gross tear film instability develops and will likely persist unless metaplasia of the lacrimal acini develops. Similarly, the toxic effect of the anti-acne drug isotretinoin on the conjunctiva surface or the meibomian glands can also result in a destabilised tear film.[13]

With the indicated use of the various drugs that can cause hypersecretion, the ADR simply has to be tolerated with judicious use of good-quality lubricating artificial tears (e.g. those with two polymers, or a higher concentration of a polymer)[24] perhaps being the most helpful. The persistent moist eyes will generally make simpler artificial tears less effective.

## Systemic medications and the cornea

Any evaluation for dry eye or infectious diseases must entail a detailed biomicroscopic examination of the cornea, with and without appropriate staining. With such scrutiny, a range of iatrogenic changes may be seen, especially in older patients who are taking a range of medications that affect the cornea. The superficial layers of the cornea can accumulate a number of drugs as a result of being photo-oxidised and any changes, as with the conjunctiva, are likely to be more evident within the palpebral aperture.

The drugs probably enter the eye via the blood–aqueous barrier and slowly permeate through the cornea, get exposed to light and form insoluble precipitates over a period of several weeks to many months. It is likely that lifestyle (exposure to the sun) plays an important role in the speed and/or extent of the precipitate formation. Occasionally these may be very visible but when an eye examination is being undertaken on a patient recently started on these medications, only microscopic traces may be evident, especially under retro-illumination.

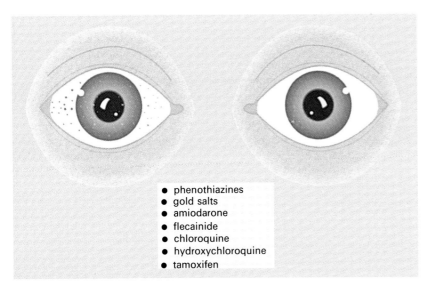

**Figure 5.7**
*Corneal deposits such as a dusting of the corneal tissue and conjunctiva (left) or forming patterns in the corneal epithelium (right).*

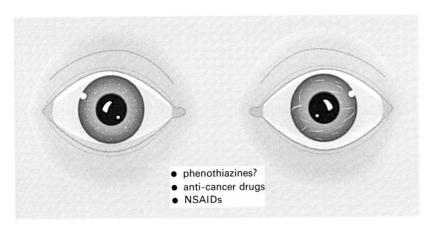

**Figure 5.8**
*Corneal surface changes (SPK) staining with fluorescein.*

For poorly understood reasons, the precipitates can simply be visible because they scatter light or develop a more obvious pale brown, golden brown or darker shades of brown to black. It should be stressed that the 'colour' of these precipitates is very much dependent upon the type of illumination used.

Perhaps the most common, when looked for, are dust-like (very small) particulate deposits in basal layer of corneal epithelium or Bowman's layer that arise in patients on neuroleptic therapy with phenothiazine drugs such as chlorpromazine or thioridazine for severe anxiety or for epilepsy (carbamazepine, Figure 5.7, left). The effect may be referred to as corneal stippling or dusting.[33-35]

Such deposits occasionally can be found deeper in the cornea and even within and across the endothelial surface, where they will more likely appear brown and need to be distinguished from true melanin deposits or bedewing. When such extensive deposits develop, episodic epitheliopathy and corneal oedema can develop.[35] Unless concurrent oedema develops, the deposits themselves are generally not associated with corneal surface staining with fluorescein unless, of course, an elderly patient suffers from some form of dry eye, perhaps resulting from drug-induced perturbation of eyeblink–tear film dynamics (see above).

However, in older patients suffering from dry eyes, a range of drugs used to manage common complaints (e.g. rheumatoid arthritis and cancer) can cause significant corneal surface changes (Figure 5.8, left).

Corneal deposits associated with epitheliopathy presenting with broken patterns or shapes and revealed as punctate and diffuse staining with fluorescein have been reported to be associated with use of high doses of some non-steroidal anti-inflammatory drugs (NSAIDs) such as oral indomethacin, oral naproxen and oral phenylbutazone[36] (Figure 5.8, right).

It is uncertain how much the appearance of such 'deposits' depends on the severity of the chronic arthritis that these drugs generally are used for. While usually rather mild, the condition could result in recurrent corneal erosion and/or increased incidence of secondary infection. The possibility of similar sorts of changes should be considered when anti-cancer drugs are being used as well as with conjunctival and tear film problems leading to the development of a toxic keratitis.[15] Other 'iatrogenic' causes should not be overlooked, e.g. topical minoxidil, or other hair-grooming oils or gels.

Another feature, but most uncommon with modern-day therapies for rheumatoid arthritis, is the possibility of discrete but refractile deposits appearing in the corneal and conjunctival epithelium without any obvious pattern being present (see Figure 5.7, left). The example here would be attributed to oral or parenteral therapy with gold salts (e.g. auranofin, sodium aurothiomalate).[9,37] Both these drugs are used as therapy for severe rheumatoid arthritis that is refractory to other drugs, but there is likely concurrent corneal disease associated with the arthritis and prior to use of NSAIDs.

Lastly, when looking at corneal epithelial deposits comes the group of drugs that can cause very distinct patterned deposits (see Figure 5.7, right). These have been widely written about for more than 30 years yet, in reality, are relatively uncommon because of the relatively low usage of these drugs and because they rarely result in corneal morbidity. These whorl-like deposits in the corneal epithelium are sometimes simply referred to as a keratopathy, 'cat's whiskers' (the author's

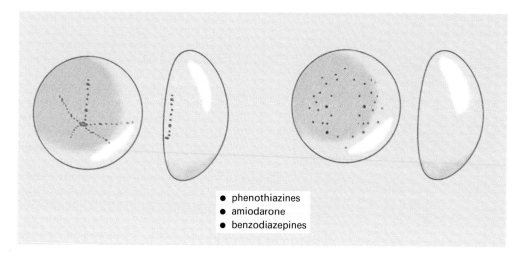

- phenothiazines
- amiodarone
- benzodiazepines

**Figure 5.9**
*Anterior lens deposits.*

preferred term) or (perhaps incorrectly) as 'corneal verticillata'.[15,38,39]

The deposits are found especially at the nasal and inferior quadrant of the cornea and just on or beyond the optic pupillary zone. Vision is unlikely to be significantly affected, although some glare can arise from dense deposits. In some cases, the deposits can be expected to develop in just a few weeks and with most patients being affected, e.g. special anti-arrhythmia drugs such as amiodarone. It should be noted that *MIMS*, for example, has simply listed the changes attributed to amiodarone as 'ophthalmic'. In other cases, despite the notoriety, these deposits can take years of therapy to develop and only affect some patients, e.g. hydroxychloroquine being used as an anti-arthritis drug, or chloroquine being used for arthritis or malaria.

For other anti-arrhythmia drugs such as flecainide, the time course for development and incidence of the changes is still uncertain,[40] although *MIMS* still lists 'rarely corneal deposits' as an ADR. While rheumatoid arthritis patients may have concurrent ocular surface disease unrelated to therapy with these drugs, the author is not aware of literature indicating corneal surface changes with, for example, hydroxychloroquine, i.e. the deposits may be spectacular but are cosmetic in that they are not likely to be associated with punctate epitheliopathy *per se*.

Perhaps more important in terms of possible corneal morbidity is the use of the anti-cancer drug tamoxifen. The pattern here can now be reminiscent of a true

corneal verticillata;[15] systemic mucopolysaccharide diseases (e.g. Fabry's) should be ruled out as a cause and concurrent epitheliopathy is more likely.

The management of corneal deposits is usually uncomplicated and rarely requires any interventive therapy. If corneal deposits develop, then these deposits on their own are not a reason for discontinuing the medication. The deposits should be monitored on a 3–6-monthly basis, depending on how intense they are and where they are. If a significant reduction (e.g. two lines) in visual acuity developed (probably due to glare and light scatter), a referral is advisable, with the intent of reducing drug dosing or discontinuation.

The use of some of the drugs (phenothiazines, tamoxifen) may also cause changes in the tear film and then produce mild symptoms (which can be managed with simple artificial tears). In rare cases, epithelial and even general corneal oedema can develop (phenothiazines). In such instances, discontinuation of the drug therapy should be arranged and the oedema should resolve over 1–2 weeks. For all cases, the deposits may slowly resolve after discontinuation of the drug, over 3–9 months.

It is important to note, however, that retinal changes can very occasionally accompany the deposits in the cornea, in which case referral and follow-up should be more aggressive. In such cases, it is more likely that the drug dosage will be reduced or the drug discontinued.

In such instances, the management

should include considerations of discontinuation (or prevention of re-exposure) of the causative agents but options in this area are limited and not usually possible with cancer therapy. Treatment should include aggressive therapy with non-preserved artificial tears; a bandage contact lens or collagen shield may help and prophylactic use of antibacterial eyedrops may be appropriate.

If there is ocular discomfort, systemic analgesics can include aspirin–codeine or paracetamol–codeine combinations rather than high-dose NSAIDs alone (i.e. ASA, paracetamol, etc) since the NSAIDs could worsen the keratitis.

## Systemic medications and the anterior crystalline lens

A number of the medications that can produce corneal deposits also appear to have the potential for producing a range of anterior lens deposits. It is possible that, in some cases, the systemic drug(s) may accumulate in the lens and be subject to photosensitisation (and thus biotransformation) before changes are evident in the cornea, although detailed pharmacokinetic data are not available.

Overall, when such drug deposits develop in the epithelium of the crystalline lens, there is no obvious link between the deposits at the two sites, i.e. a patient having pronounced corneal deposits may not have any crystalline lens deposits, and *vice versa*.

Lens epithelial deposits are uncommon nowadays although, in early stages, the deposits may be extremely difficult to see unless they are looked for; retro-illumination can be particularly useful. However, with sustained medication use, there can be a progressive development of scattered pigment deposits on or under the anterior lens capsule, that evolve to spoke-like (star-like) pigment deposits under the anterior capsule (in the lens epithelial cells) (Figure 5.9, left).

These deposits, especially if of the scattered type, may be limited to the mid-portion of the lens surface, i.e. within the natural pupil and with fewer deposits inferiorly and superiorly. Their 'colour' will very much depend upon the type of illumination used but can appear yellow-brown or grey.[7,12,34,41] Such deposits are probably irreversible and are very slowly progressive (Figure 5.9, right).

The extent of the deposits can be subjectively graded (1+, 2+, 3+, 4+) and visual acuity (VA) is not usually affected until a grade 3+ or 4+ is reached. However, less extensive deposits might just happen to be in a critical place and cause significant reduction in VA, especially if the deposits form a spoke-like arrangement and the hub of the spoke is along the visual axis.

Drugs reported to cause these types of anterior lens deposits include phenothiazine tranquillisers (e.g. oral chlorpromazine) where the spoke-like cataract usually has a dense hub, special anti-arrhythmia drugs (e.g. oral amiodarone) where either dense aggregates without obvious pattern or a spoke-like cataract can develop, and benzodiazepine tranquillisers (e.g. oral diazepam) where a general brown dusting over the lens surface can appear.[41,42]

Other systemically administered drugs, such as those for psoriasis (psoralens) or gout (allopurinol), may also photosensitise a lens but produce posterior cataract.[41]

For the most part, the development of anterior lens deposits requires nothing more than monitoring every 6–12 months. However, as with corneal deposits produced by some of these drugs (especially the phenothiazines), retinal changes can occasionally accompany the lens changes and then referral and follow-up should be more aggressive. In such cases, it is more likely that the drug dosage will be reduced or the drug discontinued.

# References

1 Doughty MJ, Rumney NK (1998) The future role of optometrists in the UK in treating anterior segment eye disease. *Optometry Today*, December 18, 33–37.

2 Kerr C, Roberson G (1995) A matter of priority. *Optician* **209**: 18–19.

3 Efron N (1997) Clinical application of grading scales for contact lens complications. *Optician* **213**: 26–35.

4 Cho P, Brown B (1993) Review of the tear break-up time and a closer look at the tear break-up time of Hong Kong Chinese. *Optom Vis Sci* **70**: 20–38.

5 Cho P, Yap M (1993) Schirmer test. I. A review. *Optom Vis Sci* **70**: 152–156.

6 Dyster-Aas K, Hansson H, Miorner G *et al.* (1974) Pigment deposits in eyes and light-exposed skin during long term methacycline therapy. *Acta Dermatol* **54**: 209–222.

7 Mathalone MBR (1967) Eye and skin changes in psychiatric patients treated with chlorpromazine. *Br J Ophthalmol* **51**: 86–93.

8 Blackstear JL, Randle HW (1991) Reversibility of blue-gray cutaneous discoloration from amiodarone. *Mayo Clin Proc* **66**: 721–726.

9 Flemming CJ, Salisbury ELC, Kirwan P *et al.* (1996) Chrysiasis after low-dose gold and UV light exposure. *J Am Acad Dermatol* **34**: 349–351.

10 Lebowitz MA, Berson DS (1988) Ocular effects of oral retinoids. *J Am Acad Dermatol* **19**: 209–211.

11 Westin EJ, Holdeman N, Perrigin D (1992) Bulbar conjunctival pigmentation secondary to oral tetracycline therapy. *Clin Eye Vision Care* **4**: 19–21.

12 Siddall JR (1966) Ocular toxic changes associated with chlorpromazine and thioridazine. *Can J Ophthalmol* **1**: 190–198.

13 Egger SF, Huber-Spitzy V, Bohler K *et al.* (1995) Ocular side effects associated with 13-cis-retinoic acid therapy for acne vulgaris: clinical features, alterations of tearfilm and conjunctival flora. *Acta Ophthalmol Scand* **73**: 355–357.

14 Burns LJ (1992) Ocular toxicities of chemotherapy. *Seminars Oncol* **19**: 492–500.

15 Al-Tweigeri T, Nabholtz J-M, Macey JR (1996) Ocular toxicity and cancer chemotherapy. *Cancer* **78**: 1359–1373.

16 Ruprecht KW, Loch EG, Giere W (1976) Sandgefühl der Augen und hormonale Kontrazeptiva. *Klin Monatsbl Augenheilkd* **163**: 198–204.

17 De Vries Reilingh A, Reiners H, Van Bijsterveld OP (1978) Contact lens tolerance and oral contraceptives. *Ann Ophthalmol (Chic)* **10**: 947–952.

18 Gurwood AS, Gurwood I, Gubman DT *et al.* (1995) Idiosyncratic ocular symptoms associated with the estradiol transdermal estrogen replacement patch system. *Optom Vis Sci* **72**: 29–33.

19 Doughty MJ, Fonn D, Richter D *et al.* (1997) A patient questionnaire approach to estimating the prevalence of dry eye symptoms in patients presenting to optometric practices across Canada. *Optom Vision Sci* **74**: 624–631.

20 Arend O, Wolf S, Harris A *et al.* (1993) Effects of oral contraceptives on conjunctival microcirculation. *Clin Hemorheol* **13**: 435–445.

21 Dollery CT, Bulpitt CJ, Daniel J, Clifton P (1977) Eye symptoms in patients taking propranolol and other hypertensive agents. *Br J Clin Pharmacol* **4**: 295–297.

22 Jachuck SJ, Stephenson J, Bird T *et al.* (1997) Practolol-induced autoantibodies and their relation to oculo-cutaneous complications. *Postgrad Med J* **53**: 75–77.

23 Severin M (1974) Keratoconjunctivitis sicca mit Bindehautschrumpfung wahrend einer Behandlung mit Dalzic. *Klin Monatsbl Augenheilkd* **165**: 941–945.

24 Doughty MJ (1997) A guide to ophthalmic pharmacy medicines in the United Kingdom. *Ophthal Physiol Opt* **17** (suppl 1): S2–S8.

25 Crandall DC, Leopold IH (1979) The influence of systemic drugs on tear constituents. *Ophthalmology* **86**: 115–125.

26 Constad WH, Bhagat N (1997) Keratitis sicca and dry eye syndrome. *Immunol Allerg Clin N America* **17**: 89–102.

27 Doughty MJ (1996) Diagnostic and therapeutic pharmaceutical agents for use in contact lens practice. In: *Clinical Contact Lens Practice* (Bennett ED, Weissman BA, eds). JB Lippincott, Philadelphia, USA Chapter 9, pp. 1–38.

28 Bergmann MT, Newman BL, Johnson NC (1985) The effect of a diuretic (hydrochlorthiazide) on tear production in humans. *Am J Ophthalmol* **99**: 473–475.

29 Koffler BH, Lemp MA (1980) The effect of an antihistamine (chlorpheniramine

maleate) on tear production in humans. *Ann Ophthalmol (Chic)* **12**: 217–219.

30 Mader TH, Stulting RD (1991) Keratoconjunctivitis sicca caused by diphenoxylate hydrocholoride with atropine sulfate (Lomotil). *Am J Ophthalmol* **111**: 377–378.

31 Mackie I A, Seal DV, Pescod JM (1977) Beta-adrenergic receptor blocking drugs: tear lysozyme and immunological screening for adverse reaction. *Br J Ophthalmol* **61**: 354–359.

32 Bagheri H, Berlan M, Montastruc JL et al. (1990) Yohimbine and lacrimal secretion (letter). *Br J Clin Pharmacol* **30**: 151–152.

33 Henderson JW, Gillespie DR (1945) An unusual type of corneal opacities. *Am J Ophthalmol* **28**: 1236–1244.

34 Alexander LJ, Bowerman L, Thompson LR (1985) The prevalence of the ocular side effects of chlorpromazine in the Tuscaloosa Veterans Administration patient population. *J Am Optom Assoc* **56**: 872–876.

35 Oshika T, Itotagawa K, Sawa M (1991) Severe corneal edema after prolonged use of psychotropic agents. *Cornea* **10**: 354–357.

36 Tillmann W, Keitel L (1977) Hornhautveranderungen durch Indometacin (Amuno). *Klin Monatsbl Augenheilkd* **170**: 756–759.

37 Bron AJ, McLendon BF, Camp V (1979) Epithelial deposition of gold in the cornea in patients receiving systemic therapy. *Am J Ophthalmol* **88**: 354–360.

38 Wilson FM, Schmitt TE, Grayson M (1980) Amiodarone-induced corneal verticillata. *Ann Ophthalmol (Chic)* **10**: 657–660.

39 Portnoy JZ, Callan JP (1983) Ophthalmologic aspects of chloroquine and hydroxychloroquine therapy. *Int J Dermatol* **18**: 273–278.

40 Moller HU, Thygesen K, Kruit PJ (1991) Corneal deposits associated with flecainide. *Br Med J* **302**: 506–507.

41 Potaznick W, Favale AF (1993) Drug-induced cataracts. *Clin Eye Vis Care* **5**: 110–116.

42 Pau H (1985) Braune scheibenformige Einlagerungen in die Linse nach Langzeitgabe von Diazepam (Valium). *Klin Monatsbl Augenheilkd* **187**: 219–220.

# 6
# Vasodilation and inflammation of the anterior surface and its management

## Introduction

The ocular surface and anterior segment of the eye are very susceptible to a wide range of 'irritants' that result in vasodilation and the development of oedema in the eyelid margins, palpebral, orbital and bulbar conjunctiva.

In the management of such conditions, it is very important that a full history and eye examination is undertaken so the different aetiologies of the presenting condition can be appreciated.[1–5]

This should include assessments of VA, pupil function, lymph nodes, direct ophthalmoscopy, slit-lamp biomicroscopy and tonometry. Binocular indirect ophthalmoscopy may still be indicated even for the apparently obvious external eye problems.

It is only from such a perspective that the appropriate management or therapy can be started, or referral arranged.

## Vasculature of the eye and its regulation

As discussed in Chapter 2, the external eye is richly supplied with blood vessels that play an important part in the delivery of drugs to the conjunctiva and the inside of the eye. The differential diagnosis of vasodilation and oedema that can develop as a result of this vasculature being 'stimulated' should consider the level at which the response occurs (Figure 6.1). Equivalent levels of vasculature also run through the palpebral conjunctiva and the stroma of the eyelids.

The initial response of the vasculature to 'irritation' is that the blood vessels dilate and, depending upon their depth, can impart varying degrees or types of blush or redness to the conjunctiva. There is reasonable evidence that the principal vasodilator is histamine in acute-onset conditions associated with external irritants and allergens, but we now know that a number of other

biological mediators are also involved in chronic vasodilation and inflammatory responses, for instance the prostaglandins and a number of small neuromodulatory peptides such as substance P.[6–8]

The actual role of the sympathetic, parasympathetic, serotoninergic and dopaminergic systems in the development of vasodilation is still a matter of some debate, but it is without any question that the histamine- and prostaglandin-mediated systems can be very effectively manipulated by topical pharmaceuticals and so reduce the vasodilation of the conjunctival vasculature and also change the anterior uveal blood flow.[4,9,10]

Sustained vasodilation results in changes in the vascular permeability such that, as a result of the fluid pressure in the vasculature, there is an ever-increasing tendency for fluid, ions and inflammatory mediators to be literally forced across the endothelial linings of the blood vessels and into the tissue. In the more superficial

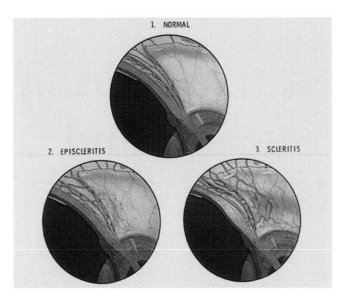

**Figure 6.1**
*The anterior vascular coat of the eye and the sites and consequences of vasodilation and oedema
from the most superficial to the deepest-lying vessels (Reproduced with permission from* Clinical
Ophthalmology. A Systematic Approach *(1999) by J. J. Kanski[1] ).*

layers of the conjunctiva, the vasodilation can obviously add to general redness and volume of the tissue and lead to the well known signs of a conjunctival blush, puffy eyelid margins and chemosis.[6,7]

The blush may involve large numbers of the relatively fine capillaries, or the response may apparently affect just a few more prominent vessels (and be referred to as an 'injection'). However, the very substantial network of blood vessels of the subepithelial tissue means that even slight extravasation can increase the volume of the bulbar conjunctiva circumferential to the cornea and it is raised slightly or substantially in acute inflammatory reactions (chemosis). These degrees of changes are readily reversible with drugs that simply constrict the dilated blood vessels.

However, in what is generally a more substantial and subacute response that develops over hours rather than minutes, a sectorial vasodilation of deeper-lying and generally coarser blood vessels results in local areas of the more peripheral bulbar conjunctiva having extremely dilated blood vessels and also being distinctly raised above the normally smooth surface, e.g. as in episcleritis.

A slightly different response occurs as the deepest blood vessels are involved. Here, the entire bulbar (and orbital) conjunctiva and sclera can be expected to become extre-

mely sensitive to touch and be painful as the tissue is distended due to deep lying oedema. The magnitude and reason for this response can be considered as a simple consequence of the size (bore) of the blood vessels involved for, as clearly evident in scleritis, deeper lying and generally coarser blood vessels (that have a less prominent redness) are involved.

As part of the history and differential diagnosis, different types of internal causes of superficial and deeper-lying vasodilation need to be ruled out (Table 6.1).

For superficial changes, these are related

to trauma and infection, while for deeper-lying reactions, the main causes are related to inflammation arising within the anterior uveal tissue (iritis and anterior uveitis) and vasodilation arising from subacute elevation of intraocular pressure (angle-closure glaucoma).

Remarkable and gross vasodilation can be evident across the bulbar conjunctiva that can distract attention from the deeper lying blood vessels. However, the accompanying pupillary and corneal signs should usually prove adequate for a correct diagnosis to be made.[1,5]

## Palliative management options – eyewashes and cold compresses

Acute irritation of the surface of the eye by allergens or some chemical substances can lead to watery eyes, puffy eyelid margins and chemosis (Figure 6.2); there may be a general hyperaemia as well. The history here will often be exposure to plant or animal allergens,[9,10] but it is important that such a response is differentiated from a watery eye associated with a mechanical irritation (e.g. an inwardly pointing eyelash, Figure 6.3) or an embedded corneal or conjunctival foreign body (see later) or a viral or chlamydial infection.

Part of the management of this type of allergic conjunctivitis is to reduce the levels of the offending irritant from the ocular surface after the eye examination by use of an eyewash (e.g. plastic ampoules of Vital Eyes, or sterile saline such as GSL Steri-Wash or GSL Steripod Blue) or an

---

**Table 6.1   Important considerations in the differential diagnosis of red eyes**

- History of development of the red or pink eye
- Workplace, home and environment
- Any coexisting systemic disease?
- Any concurrent eyelid margin disease?
- Any obvious causative agents (allergens, etc)?
- Any iatrogenic causes (medications)?
- Nature of any discharge/lacrimation?
- Any evidence of tear film dysfunction?
- Any foreign body?
- Any pupil anomaly or dysfunction?
- Any accompanying corneal disease?
- What is the depth of the vasodilation?
- Any anterior chamber reaction?
- Do the symptoms include pain (rather than discomfort)?
- Any concurrent infection(s)?

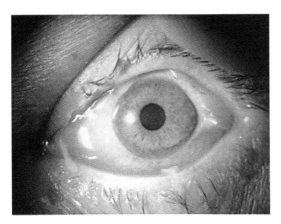

**Figure 6.2**
*Watery eyes, puffy eyelid margins and chemosis associated with allergic conjunctivitis (Reproduced with permission from* Clinical Ophthalmology. A Systematic Approach *(1999) by J. J. Kanski[1]).*

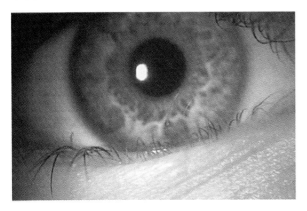

**Figure 6.3**
*Watery eyes and mild conjunctival blush associated with an inward pointing eyelash (Reproduced with permission from* Clinical Ophthalmology. A Systematic Approach *(1999) by J. J. Kanski[1]).*

## Cleansing options – lid scrubs and astringents

The presentation of a conjunctival blush and eyelid margin redness and oedema may also be associated with the persistent presence of natural secretions, exogenous irritants, or bacterial toxins on the eyelid margins (Figure 6.4). The condition can be associated with moderate but persistent allergic reactions, but other causes such as a generally poor facial hygiene, mild meibomian gland congestion or mild bacterial infections also need to be considered.

In all cases, while a little more attention to hygiene can be effective, the condition is best managed with more than just a simple eye wash.[9–11] Starting a once-daily cleansing of the eyelid margins with a commercial lid scrub product (e.g. Lid Care solution or sterile wipes) (Figure 6.5) will both remove the sebaceous or oily secretions and collarettes from the eyelashes, as well as promote meibomian gland expression – largely a result of the gentle eyelid massage that results from the cleansing procedure.

The commercial products, applied with either a clean gauze cloth or a clean cotton bud applicator, are designed to replace baby shampoo.[10,11] While it might be argued that any attention to lid hygiene is better than none, attempts to cleanse the eyelid margin with a face flannel dabbed in a shampoo product has to be questioned not only on the grounds of efficacy, but also patient satisfaction and compliance; use of a commercial product is more likely to produce useful results.

astringent (e.g. GSL Optrex products; see below).[10,11] The eyelid oedema and chemosis can be reduced by placing an ice cube in a clean gauze pad over the closed eye for a few minutes; a clean face flannel or tea-towel pre-soaked in cold tap water is an alternative. The procedure may be repeated 15 minutes later.

While the condition is self-limiting and will resolve in an hour or so without intervention, the use of the eye wash and the cold 'compress' serves to augment the body's natural response (reflex lacrimation) to wash out the irritant and to constrict the superficial blood vessels that have responded to the allergen and produced the acute oedema of both the eyelid margins and the bulbar conjunctiva.

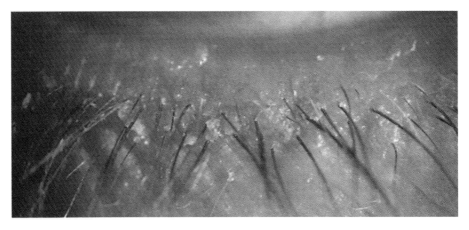

**Figure 6.4**
*Slightly watery eyes, reddened and puffy eyelid margins with conjunctival hyperaemia, associated with low grade blepharitis (Reproduced with permission from* Clinical Ophthalmology. A Systematic Approach *(1999) by J. J. Kanski[1]).*

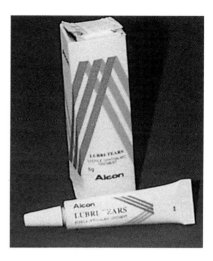

**Figure 6.5**
*Commercial products for cleansing the eyelids.*

In addition to lid margin hygiene, the eye may respond well to regular cleansing with an astringent (e.g. GSL Optrex Eye Lotion, supplied with an eye-cup, see Chapter 4). After cleansing, a drop of astringent eyedrops (e.g. GSL Optrex Eye Drops, Optrex Fresh Eyes, Vital Eyes drops or P Zinc Sulphate eye drops, see Chapter 4) can also promote comfort, especially if the eyelid cleansing was a little too aggressive. Patients should be instructed to carry out a programme of cleansing for a definite period, e.g. 2 or 4 weeks and then be reviewed to ensure both compliance and efficacy.

## Supportive measures – artificial tears

In cases of blepharitis, patients may be mildly symptomatic and have slight con-

junctival hyperaemia as a result of tear film instability,[1,2,10] and thus may benefit from periodic tear film replacement using a simple artificial tears product.[11] Similarly, if the eyelid margins have been cleaned, the normal tear film is disrupted and the use of an eyedrop should promote comfort as well as supplement the tear film as it is re-established.

This can be very important since if there is a tear film deficiency (leading to 'dry eyes'), or any other reason why patients' tears will not form a stable film across the surface of the eye, slight superficial vasodilation can result. Causes can be the inadequate formation of the lower tear film meniscus in milder cases of ectropion, inadequate eyelid closure leading to exposure (Figure 6.6), as well as general lacrimal hyposecretion. The causes of the hyposecretion or poor tear film quality can be disease,[12] or simply associated with systemic medication use (Chapter 5).

The 'as-needed' (*prn*) use of a simple artificial tear[11,12] can substantially increase patient comfort and indirectly reduce the vasodilation simply because the persistent irritant (the unstable tear film) is attenuated. If the dry eyes were due to systemic medication, regular use of the artificial tears an hour or so after taking the medications may be much more effective than an 'as-needed' schedule.

In these types of conditions, there is rarely a need for high-polymer lubricating artificial tears or gel lubricants, nor ophthalmic ointments. However, patients should be considered on an individual

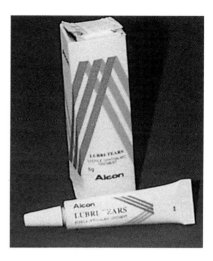


**Figure 6.7**
*Topical unmedicated ophthalmic ointment (P medicine) containing white paraffin and lanolin.*

basis for a definitive case of lagophthalmos may respond well to the nightly (*od*) use of unmedicated and unpreserved ophthalmic ointments.

The principal constituent can be soft white paraffin (e.g. P Lubritears, Figure 6.7) or soft yellow paraffin (e.g. P Simple Eye Ointment, Figure 6.8). A white paraffin product is likely also to contain lanolin to ensure uniform texture. Similarly, more severe cases of lacrimal disease or medication-related dry eyes may also need ocular lubricants[1-4,12] or even punctal occlusion.[13]

## Countering vasodilation – ocular decongestants and antihistamine eyedrops

Any time there is mild but chronic irritation of the external eye, there is likely to be a vasodilatory response evident across the bulbar conjunctiva that is not associated with substantial lacrimation. A history of exposure to a dry or dusty working environment, exposure to chemical fumes (in the workplace or at home), or working or leisure practices that lead to excessive eye strain can also be associated with mild conjunctival vasodilation. All of these conditions can be managed with ophthalmic decongestants *prn*.

However, there are other aetiologies that should also be considered and where there

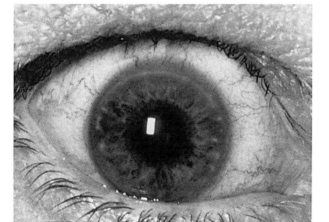

**Figure 6.6**
*Mild vasodilation associated with excessive exposure of the superior conjunctiva, associated with eyelid retraction (Reproduced with permission from* Clinical Ophthalmology. A Systematic Approach *(1999) by J. J. Kanski[1]).*

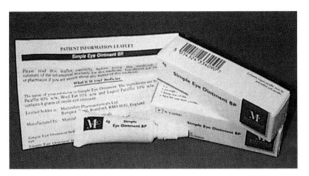

**Figure 6.8**
*Topical unmedicated and lanolin-free ophthalmic ointment (P medicine) containing yellow paraffin.*

is perhaps a greater risk of inappropriate use of decongestants for different reasons; these include inadequate tear production or inadequate tear coverage (see above) or the wearing of a contact lens (see below). In addition, it is important to avoid trying to manage an angry-looking eye with decongestants when the cause is an abrasion or a foreign body. These causes should all be assumed when one is presented with a red eye – until ruled out by examination.

Such trauma can be easy to detect when it is on the corneal surface, yet could equally well be buried under the eyelids and within a chemotic palpebral conjunctiva. Hence, lid eversion is an essential part of the eye examination (which may be facilitated by judicious use of a topical ocular anaesthetic and even perhaps a drop of decongestant). Such trauma-associated vasodilation may need substantially more management than decongestants (see Chapter 9).

Ophthalmic decongestants or ocular antihistamines are meant to provide occasional relief of symptoms associated with mildly irritated eyes and to improve the cosmetic appearance of the external eye, eyelid margins, etc. This relief should be attempted only two to three times daily. All too often these reasons are reversed and the products are used to 'whiten' eyes that really only need a good wash, reduction in contact lens wear or even just a little sleep; every 2 hours or more than six times a day should be considered as excessive or overuse.

It is thus important to ascertain the cause of the irritation rather than just use eyedrops. This includes consideration of whether there is a genuine allergic component, in which case oral antihistamines

and mast-cell stabilisers may be more appropriate (see below). Similarly, for dirt, dust and irritating vapours, a good eye wash could achieve excellent results.

It is also important to note that excessive use of these decongestant products, especially if there is continuing irritation (e.g. swimming pools, petrol fumes, dry eyes, etc) can lead to a rebound effect in which the condition both becomes relatively refractory to the vasoconstrictive action of the decongestants and the vasculature redilates 4–6 hours later to a greater level than before.[9,14]

Symptoms do not necessarily get worse when the rebound signs appear. Largely anecdotal evidence suggests that these types of products could also actually reduce the ocular sensitivity to allergens and irritants. The question here is whether there could be a prophylactic effect in that the extent of a cycle of hyperaemia/injection/mild oedema, etc, could be reduced by prior instillation of these eyedrops.

If there is such prophylactic efficacy, it is more likely the result of slight reflex lacrimation (precipitated by the eyedrops) that serves as a mini eye wash (see section on mast-cell stabilisers).

Topical ocular decongestants are undoubtedly effective 'eye whiteners' and a self-medication to manage an eye with acute or subacute mild foreign-body sensation, gritty feelings, etc, as well as the 'pain across the front of my eyes' from a day in the sun, at the beach, pool, etc. However, as part of the history and eye examination, it should be remembered that these decongestants can be equally effective in masking other problems and that they are not the 'cure-all' for all types of irritated eyes.

Since these products are frequently used in the belief that they are effective as prophylactic as well as treatment drugs (see below), it is important to establish if a patient has been using these types of products and, if possible, ask them to refrain from using them for a day before the examination.

The decongestant activity is the result of direct alpha-adrenergic action or histamine $H_1$-blocking action on the more superficial conjunctival vasculature. Both types of drugs, especially the adrenergics, will either attenuate vasodilation or cause vasoconstriction – thus the term 'decongestants'. The adrenergic drugs used in these products are primarily considered to interact directly with $alpha_1$-receptors on the blood vessels of the conjunctiva and cause vasoconstriction. There is some evidence, however, that $alpha_2$-type receptors are also present in conjunctival tissue (including the blood vessels) and antihistamines also probably work through a range of receptors, on both the conjunctiva and eyelid margins.

For either, drug interaction with the receptors will help counter vasodilation and also the other signs and symptoms of a mild inflammatory reaction. The other signs and symptoms include discomfort, puffiness/oedema (chemosis) and reflex lacrimation, and all will probably be attenuated by use of the decongestant or antihistamine.[9]

If the products also contain an antihistamine ($H_1$-blocking), additional efficacy against itchiness symptoms can be expected. All these products contain preservatives (usually benzalkonium chloride and edetate sodium).

A range of multi-use (10 ml) eyedrop products, such as P medicines, are usually available in the UK.[10,11] They include phenylephrine 0.12% as an $alpha_1$-adrenergic (e.g. P Isopto Frin, Figure 6.9). Naphazoline 0.01% as an $alpha_1$-adrenergic combined with an astringent such as witch-hazel 12% is also available (e.g. P Eye Dew, see Chapter 4) and naphazoline 0.01–0.1% in eyedrops in combination with a histamine $H_1$-blocker such as antazoline (e.g. P Murine), xylometazoline 0.05% as an adrenergic (with both $alpha_1$ and $alpha_2$ actions) in combination products with an antihistamine antazoline (e.g. P Otrivine–Antistin, see Chapter 4). Also available is a topical antihistamine on

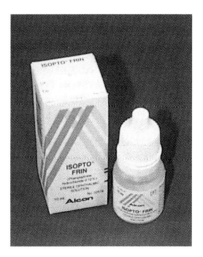

**Figure 6.9**
*Topical decongestant (P medicine) for short-term, occaisional use in conjunctivitis associated with general irritation, allergens, tired eyes, etc.*

its own, i.e. levocabastine 0.05% as P Livostin Direct (Figure 6.10).

Eye whiteners can promptly relieve acute-onset symptoms and greatly improve the cosmetic appearance of the external eye. For their safe and effective clinical use, a number of things should be considered related primarily to systemic medical concerns and the long-term health of the cornea and conjunctiva.

The use of these products containing alpha$_1$-adrenergic decongestants is contraindicated (C/I) in narrow-angle glaucoma – a listed ADR (e.g. in *MIMS*) is angle-closure and such an ADR has been reported.[9,11] These products should

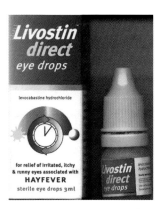

**Figure 6.10**
*Topical antihistamine (P Medicine) for occasional use in conjunctivitis associated with allergens.*

therefore only be recommended with care, or given to elderly patients if the intraocular pressure or outflow facility/angles, etc, are known. These products should not generally be recommended/provided to patients with substantial blood pressure disorders, cardiac disorders, or a history of stroke or hyperthyroidism, or if pregnant. The ocular decongestant eyedrops should thus be treated as if they were all phenylephrine.

For example, patients with inadequate tear film maintenance due to lid retraction-associated hyperthyroid disorders should not overuse such products. In this case, the decongestants could exacerbate the condition (perhaps even by marginally further widening the palpebral aperture), and tear film supplementation would likely be a better option in this case. The point here is that the concentration of the vasoconstrictors may be small but, with overuse, systemic effects can occur.

Packaging or inserts for these products often carry such warnings and may also include (labile) diabetes on the list of diseases. It is not that these products contain high concentrations of dangerous drugs, but simply that they can be easily overused and many drops can produce a higher dose.

The same types of precautions also apply to use of nasal decongestants (e.g. P Otrivine Nasal Drops or P Sudafed nasal sprays containing oxymetazoline). Just as the history-taking should include consideration of systemic diseases, there is also a need for a complete medications history (see Chapter 1).

There are certain interactions (INT) and specific precautions (S/P) for concurrent medications when the use of ophthalmic decongestants and antihistamines is being considered.[10,11] For example, the packaging is likely to state that the use of these products should be carefully supervised in patients taking monoamine oxidase inhibitors (MAOI). By extension and clinical reporting of adverse drug reactions, this precaution should also extend to the entire range of indirect-acting sympathomimetic or indirect-acting serotoninergic drugs, e.g. RIMAs, SNRIs, SSRIs (see Chapter 3). This is a rapidly changing area of medication use and now also includes the noradrenaline reuptake inhibitor (NARI) reboxetine,[15] and the noradrenaline and specific serotonin antidepressant (NaSSA) mirtazapine.[16]

The main risk when these are used with topical decongestants is of systemic sympathomimetic effects, consequential to unavoidable systemic absorption via the conjunctiva (see Chapter 2). However, the product labels for the ophthalmic decongestants may simply carry a statement concerning the concurrent use of anti-depressants.

It is now commonplace for pharmaceutical directories to contain a note under contraindications (C/I) about contact lens wear. In the author's opinion, this is an unfortunate contradiction that can often lead to longer-term unnecessary ocular morbidity (rather than decreasing it). What the manufacturers and CSM are trying to communicate is that they do not want patients to be instilling these eyedrops – to help maintain contact lens wear – while the offending lenses that are causing discomfort are actually in place.

That some manufacturers actually stipulate 'soft' contact lenses provides the reason for the concern in that a minority of individuals have managed to communicate a view that the preservatives in decongestant eyedrops could actually cause epithelial disease. That preservative-containing vasoconstrictors have been advocated and/or used for so many years concurrent with contact lens wear without major sequelae has not obviously been taken into account.[9]

Preservative-containing eyedrops may have to be used with bandage contact lenses (simply because suitable preservative-free products are not available in a particular situation, or at an institution) and thus in eyes with an epitheliopathy already present.[9] The issue and relevance of the warning here, which is also relevant to nasal decongestants that contain preservatives, is one of inappropriate overuse, i.e. an attempted management of a genuine contact lens intolerance,[17] or developing infection (see below). There has been no obvious and case-history supported detailed documentation to argue against the occasional use of topical decongestants to quieten the bulbar conjunctiva of an eye slightly irritated by either soft contact lens wear or moderately irritated by RGP lens wear, especially if the lenses are taken out briefly (and rinsed), the eyedrops instilled and the lenses re-inserted some 5 minutes later.

Precautionary notes are now changing to a more user-friendly perspective, e.g. 'Do

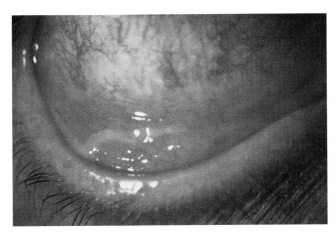

**Figure 6.11**
*Mild bulbar and palpebral vasodilation associated with mild bacterial conjunctivitis; the accompanying mucopurulent discharge in the lower fornix should be noted. This eye should not be managed solely with decongestants, although they may provide additional symptomatic relief concurrent with antibacterial drugs (Reproduced with permission from* Clinical Ophthalmology. A Systematic Approach *(1999) by J. J. Kanski[1]).*

only more important but also more complicated (Figures 6.12 and 6.13).

The first case represents those types of enteroviral or adenoviral conjunctivitis where part of the initial supportive management can include the use of cold compresses and sparing use of topical decongestants to promote conjunctival vasoconstriction and make the eye more comfortable (although systemic analgesics will also often be still needed, see Chapter 8).

The second case is an allergic reaction but not of the type associated with seasonal allergens, etc. This case results from a severe systemic cell-mediated allergic response (Figure 6.13) for which urgent referral for topical and possibly systemic treatment with corticosteroids is essential (see Chapter 9). In either case, it will be the history that should provide the clues to the aetiology of the condition,

not use whilst or immediately before wearing contact lenses'.[17] The 'immediately' before can be reliably translated to 5 minutes in many cases.[17,18]

Ophthalmic decongestants (and antihistamines) should not be used to try to manage an infected eye, or one perceived at risk of developing an infection, even though this may be a common reason for abuse of such products. They may well be used in an attempt to provide relief of symptoms and reduce signs in developing eye infection (Figure 6.11); the accompanying mucopurulent discharge in the lower fornix should be noted. This eye should not be solely managed with decongestants, although these may provide additional symptomatic relief concurrent with the use of antibacterial drugs (see Chapter 8).

That decongestants should not be used to try to manage an eye infection is the primary reason why most of these types of products carry a warning to the effect that a physician should be consulted if irritation persists for more than a few days. It is for this reason also that one should try to avoid excessive use of these products in young children where mild bacterial infections (pink eye) can be commonplace.

Beyond being useful as an adjunct therapy in mild bacterial conjunctivitis or blepharoconjunctivitis, there are some other uses for topical ocular decongestants (and antihistamines) in ocular infections, although the differential diagnosis is not

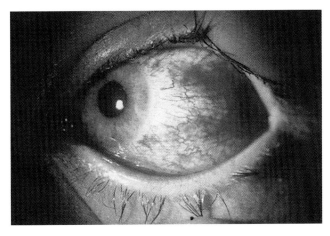

**Figure 6.12**
*Viral conjunctivitis of the epidemic type due to enterovirus or adenovirus (Reproduced with permission from* Clinical Ophthalmology. A Systematic Approach *(1999) by J. J. Kanski[1]).*

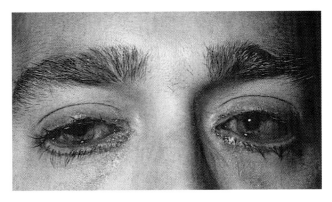

**Figure 6.13**
*Severe (cell-mediated) allergic conjunctivitis in Stevens-Johnson syndrome (Reproduced with permission from* Clinical Ophthalmology. A Systematic Approach *(1999) by J. J. Kanski[1]).*

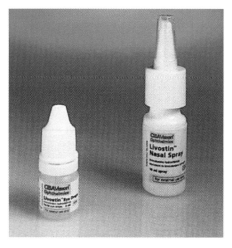

**Figure 6.14**
*Topical antihistamine for medium-term use in type I allergic conjunctivitis (with its companion product of allergic rhinitis).*

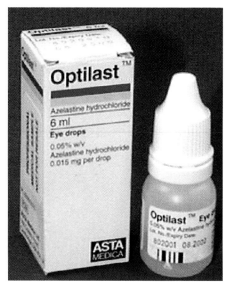

**Figure 6.15**
*Topical antihistamine for long-term use in seasonal allergic conjunctivitis.*

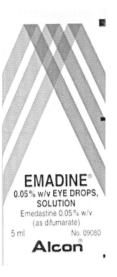

**Figure 6.16**
*Topical antihistamine for long-term use in seasonal allergic conjunctivitis.*

rather than these simply being treated as yet another red eye (and the patient being inappropriately prescribed chloramphenicol and betamethasone eyedrops).

As noted earlier, in addition to trauma (abrasions or foreign bodies), there are two other types of substantial vasodilation that should not be overlooked in the differential diagnosis. These are the acute, sometimes gross, and often circumcorneal vasodilation that can accompany the onset of either iritis (see Chapter 9) or the angle-closure form of glaucoma (see Table 6.1).[4]

As indicated above, topical ocular antihistamines are generally not recommended for long-term use, mainly because these P medications are marketed in combination with a decongestant. However, for some chronic sufferers of allergic conjunctivitis, newer options are available in the form of levocabastine 0.05% eyedrops both as P Livostin Direct (Figure 6.10) and POM Livostin (Figure 6.14). This H$_1$-blocker appears to be able to manage more chronic conditions in that it does attenuate the severity of the signs and symptoms.[9,10,19] At this time, it is recommended, however, that use should not exceed one month so it should not be used for the duration of the allergy season. It is also not recommended for use in children (under the age of 12 years or 9 years depending on whether it is the P or POM product).

Notwithstanding these limitations to its use, efficacy evaluations indicate that the action of levocabastine can be expected to be longer than other decongestants or

combinations, and so it can be used just twice daily (*bd*), as well as three times a day (*tds*) or four times a day (*qds*), depending on severity of the condition.

At this time, substantiative data are not really available on long-term efficacy for different schedules of levocabastine use.

Two other topical antihistamines are also available for use in seasonal allergic conjunctivitis.[20,21] The first is azelastine 0.05% (POM Optilast) (Figure 6.15) and the second is emedastine 0.05% (POM Emadine) (Figure 6.16). Neither is recommended for use in really young children, but there are no imposed limits on the duration of the treatment period during the allergy season.

## Countering vasodilation – oral antihistamines

Conjunctival vasodilation, lacrimation and symptoms of discomfort can often develop due to allergic causes and thus often be accompanied by systemic symptoms, i.e. nasal congestion or a runny nose. In such cases, and where the problem is more occasional than persistent, the use of oral histamine H$_1$-blockers (oral antihistamines) can be very beneficial.

In more severe but predictable chronic cases of allergic conjunctivitis (or rhino-conjunctivitis), systemic administration of these antihistamines is generally

indicated.[4,10,22] Prescription-only medications will generally only be needed if there are significant and chronic nasal, upper-respiratory or dermatological signs and symptoms accompanying any (blepharo) conjunctivitis.

Patient instructions on the use of selected pharmacy medicines in this category is thus a very useful option for the management of allergic conjunctivitis. However, it is important to remember that considerations of medical and medications history are also important here. These oral antihistamines have some sympathomimetic potential, so their use in patients with known cardiac disease, significant blood pressure disorders or any disorder that might predispose them to cardiac arrhythmias is not recommended.

Concurrent administration of other drugs with sympathomimetic potential (MAO inhibitors, etc) should be done cautiously. None of these oral antihistamine drugs are generally recommended for children, although they can be administered at half the adult dosing.

Current recommendations also limit their use in patients with epilepsy, mainly because of the potential for drug–drug interactions between their medications and the antihistamines (see Chapter 3).

Current products include chlorpheniramine (e.g. P Calimal or P Piriton, available in blister packs of 30 tablets each containing 4 mg); acrivastine (e.g. Benadryl Allergy Relief), clemastine (e.g. P Aller-Eze, available in blister packs of 10 or 30 tablets each containing 1.34 mg), and cetirizine (e.g. P Zirtek, available in blister packs of seven tablets of 10 mg each).

Some of these products may be only indicated for once-daily use (e.g. cetirizine), while others (chlorpheniramine, acrivastine and clemastine) can be used *bds* or even *qds*. All that is needed is enough systemic antihistamine to reduce symptoms and signs to an acceptable level, so the doses used do not have to produce systemic side-effects such as drowsiness, etc.

There are many other systemic antihistamines available and while they may help relieve some ocular symptoms, they are more generally indicated for other purposes, e.g. as nasal antihistamines and decongestants.

Two other oral antihistamines, terfenadine and astemizole, were available as P Medicines (e.g. P Hismanal, P Pollen-Eze, P Triludan, P Aller-Eze Clear, P Seldane). These reverted to POM status as a result of inappropriate over-use precipitating an unacceptable incidence of ADRs. A general warning for a potentially serious ADR when using terfenadine was issued in the UK in 1994 and eventually led to a specific contraindication (C/I) that it should not be taken concurrently with a range of oral antibiotics (e.g. erythromycin, ketoconazole, itraconazole) or with processed grapefruit juice.

The anti-infective drugs and the grapefruit juice were found substantially to reduce the rate of biotransformation of terfenadine and thus its bioelimination, with the result that a patient effectively over-dosed with even standard dosing. At high doses, terfenadine was found to precipitate cardiac arrhythmias and these have proved fatal in a very few cases.[23] Both drugs have now been withdrawn from general use.

A comprehensive medications history is obviously very important. For all oral antihistamines, current awareness and consideration of patients' 'right to know' mean that it should also be ascertained whether the intended patient is pregnant or breast feeding.

## Countering vasodilation – mast-cell stabilisers

The management of seasonal allergic conjunctivitis, vernal (kerato) conjunctivitis and several forms of papillary

conjunctivitis cannot be achieved with cold compresses, eyewashes, decongestants and direct-acting antihistamines alone; drugs which actually reduce the release of histamine are needed.[4,9,10]

It is important that this special aspect of the management of vasodilation is recognised. It has been advocated that topical decongestants could reduce the severity of irritative conjunctivitis if used immediately before an anticipated exposure to a mild irritant or allergen. It should be recognised, however, that these products generally sting somewhat on instillation, briefly stimulating tear flow which could also prompt wash-out of irritants. Water or a cold-compress could thus be similarly effective in relieving symptoms.

A type of prophylactic efficacy can be expected from oral antihistamines simply because they can provide symptomatic relief over a few hours in the face of continuing allergen exposure as a result of the expected pharmacokinetics of the drugs. However, the efficacy of any of the topical decongestants or antihistamines as prophylactic agents is questionable and none of them should be overused in an attempt to quell substantial ocular symptoms.

Therefore, for 'simple' chronic cases of allergic conjunctivitis, with minimal systemic involvement, topical mast-cell stabilisers can and should be used.

It has been estimated that some 10–15% of the population has chronic symptomatic atopic diseases, with seasonal allergic conjunctivitis and irritative conjunctivitis being the most common of these diseases. When the ocular involvement is substantial, it can include marked vasodilation, chronic oedema of the lid margins and conjunctiva, along with infiltrates accompanied by a high level of discomfort and foreign-body sensation. In such cases, all of the above treatment(s), and even local corticosteroid treatment for the eyelid margins and palpebral conjunctiva may also be necessary (see Chapter 9).

Medications for the nasal (e.g. Figure 6.14) and respiratory tract may also be indicated, so the patient is either already being seen by a general practitioner or should be referred for assessment. Management of any chronic cases in young children or infants should also be carried out by a general medical practitioner.

The term 'mast-cell stabilisers' is actually a non-medical one of limited scientific use simply because some or perhaps all of these

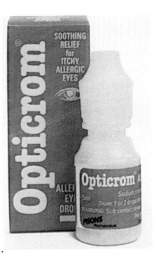

**Figure 6.17**
*Topical mast-cell stabiliser (P medicine) for initial use in chronic type I allergic conjunctivitis.*

drugs clearly do more than simply stop the conjunctival mast cells from releasing histamine. The overall result of treatment with these drugs is to reduce the release of histamine and other allergic reaction-producing chemicals and to reduce the reactions of the white blood cells to the allergens.

There are three drugs available in the UK with such indirect histamine-blocking actions.[9,10] The most well-known products contain sodium cromoglycate 2% eyedrops (alternatively known as disodium cromoglycate, cromolyn sodium or cromolyn, and to be renamed sodium cromoglicate), e.g. P Opticrom Allergy Eye Drops (Figure 6.17), P Optrex Hayfever Allergy Eye Drops, P Hay-crom Hayfever Eye Drops, P Boots Hayfever Relief Allergy Eye Drops (see Chapter 4, Figure 4.9), POM Opticrom Eye Drops, POM Cusilyn Eye Drops, POM Hay-crom Eye Drops, POM Vividrin Eye Drops, POM Viz-On Eye Drops and several POM generic products.

The difference between those bottles available as P Medicines and those as POM products is simply the size. A P medicine is usually available as a 5 ml (or perhaps a 10 ml) bottle for short-term, initial management of allergic conjunctivitis. It is the POM product, however, that should be used for chronic conditions since a few bottles, prescribed one at a time, should last the season and be very cost-effective.

For management of vernal conjunctivitis, both the eyedrops and an

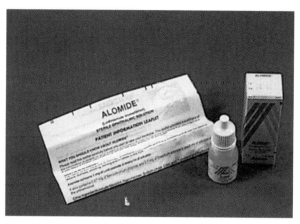

**Figure 6.18**
*Topical mast-cell stabiliser (POM) for long-term use in chronic type I allergic conjunctivitis.*

ophthalmic ointment containing 4% sodium cromoglycate (POM Opticrom) should be used (with the ointment for *od* application). Newer topical mast-cell stabilisers include lodoxamide 0.1% ophthalmic solution (POM Alomide, Figure 6.18) and nedocromil sodium 2% eyedrops (POM Rapitil, see Chapter 4, Figure 4.16).

The mast-cell stabilisers are not 'cure-all' products and their effective use requires consideration of several things, beyond whether the patient has any other forms of allergy and/or whether they have used one of these drugs previously (although it can be noted that, to date, the number of allergic-type reactions for sodium cromoglycate products has been extraordinarily small).

These drugs are indicated for prophylactic use to offset the severity of ocular reactions to allergens rather than being indicated for the provision of short-term or acute relief. It may take a week or so for the maximum protective effect to be realised and even then this may only be a substantial reduction in symptoms rather than complete suppression of symptoms in the continuing presence of the allergens; patients may have good days and bad days.

In the initial period of therapy, and for the 'bad days', topical ocular decongestants/antihistamines (e.g. P Otrivine-Antistine), the use of eyebaths with astringents (e.g. GSL Optrex Eye Lotion) and cold compresses may not only be needed but should be recommended. The goal is to maintain a quiet eye free of the 'itchy burnies' and lacrimation.[9–11]

In order for these drugs to have a reasonable chance of realising a full efficacy, it is important to recognise that dosing needs to be regular and continuous, e.g. every 4 or 6 hours (*q4h* or *q6h*) depending on severity of the condition, or the estimate of the allergen levels anticipated, and should be every day. Patients appear to be able to tolerate sodium cromoglycate eyedrops for extended periods of time (i.e. months) without a significant reduction in the sensitivity to the drug or adverse reactions occurring,[9,10] and it appears likely that the same can be expected for the other two mast-cell stabilisers as well.

However, at least for POM Opticrom or equivalent, if a higher dosing (e.g. every 3 hours (*q3h*)) is considered useful for a few days, the patient should be advised that the recommended upper dosing limit is 16 drops per day per eye. If this level of dosing is not effective, supplementary medications are needed.

Similarly, recommendations for the newer mast-cell stabilisers (lodoxamide and nedocromil sodium) advise that their continuous use should not exceed several weeks. Since the dosing needs to be regular, patient education is important and the verbal and written instructions to the patient should stress this regular use.

Sodium cromoglycate, and probably lodoxamide and nedocromil sodium, can also be used to manage vernal conjunctivitis and other chronic allergic conditions affecting the conjunctiva, although neither of the two newer drugs are currently recommended for use in younger children. However, when used, the dosing really needs to be regular (*qds*), and sustained.

Another use, at least for POM sodium cromoglycate eyedrops, is as part of the management of contact lens-induced giant papillary conjunctivitis. While the scientific logic may be questionable because the offending 'irritant' should have been removed before mast-cell stabiliser therapy started,[9] a short course (2–4 weeks) on a *qds* basis has a remarkable efficacy at resolving GPC,[4,9] and thus sparing the eye periodic corticosteroid therapy (see below).

A still very contentious issue is whether a mast-cell stabiliser should be used concurrently with contact lens wear.[9] Just as one can find the sternest criticism for the use of topical ocular decongestants while maintaining a contact lens wear schedule, there will be similar critics of such a use of mast-cell stabilisers (where the scientific logic is now surely acceptable because the contact lens wear continues). However, the same issue of a soft contact lens acting as a reservoir for the preservative (e.g. benzalkonium chloride) in the eyedrops and thus putting the corneal epithelium at risk for an iatrogenic effect still appears to guide the regulatory agencies. Contact lens wear and concurrent use of a mast-cell stabiliser is thus not recommended. This must absolutely apply to nedocromil sodium eyedrops, which have a distinct canary yellow coloration.

However, a case surely cannot be made that a contact lens-wearing eye cannot be maintained in a lesser inflammatory state by regular and concurrent sodium cromoglycate 2% eyedrop use, providing the contact lenses are removed for brief periods (see above).

## Countering vasodilation – corticosteroids and NSAIDs

Corticosteroids and non-steroidal anti-inflammatory drugs have been developed for the management of seasonal and vernal conjunctivitis, as well as for the management of other types of more serious inflammation, including that occurring after ocular surgery (see Chapter 9). It is very important to note the current indications for use of products containing these drugs in the UK.

Notwithstanding, it can be noted here that in severe cases of seasonal, vernal and giant papillary conjunctivitis, short courses (*qds* dosing, 1–3 weeks' duration) of topical corticosteroid treatment may well be needed to reduce the severity of the conditions and/or promote initial resolution.[4,9]

In North America, some NSAIDs are indicated for use in the short- and longer-term management of the vasodilation and inflammation in these diseases and also enjoy widespread use as postoperative 'steroid-sparing' drugs in the UK, Europe and North America.

Both the corticosteroids and NSAIDs counter the vasodilation and the mechanisms underlying the margination and emigration of the inflammatory cells and so are not generally indicated for the types of inflammatory reaction dealt with in this module. However, oral NSAIDs such as acetyl salicylic acid, ibuprofen and flurbiprofen can be used for their analgesic efficacy to manage the pain associated with inflammation of the conjunctiva.[1,2]

## Conclusions

By our current understanding, vasodilation and the ensuing oedema of the conjunctiva and eyelid margins is principally mediated through the actions of histamine. The priorities for the therapeutic management of such conditions involves removing the offending stimuli (by irrigation or cleansing), ensuring adequate tear film coverage of the ocular surface and using a range of drugs to counter the vasodilation in either the short or long term.

These drugs need to be carefully selected according to the type of condition being managed and taking into account the expected duration and clinical course of the inflammatory processes.

## References

1 Kanski JJ (1999) *Clinical Ophthalmology. A Systematic Approach*, 4th edn. Butterworth-Heinemann, Oxford, UK.

2 Kanski JJ, Nischal KK (1999) *Ophthalmology. Clinical Signs and Differential Diagnosis*. Mosby, London.

3 Okhravi N (1997) *Manual of Primary Eye Care*. Butterworth-Heinemann, Oxford, UK.

4 Crick RP, Knaw PT (1997) *A Textbook of Clinical Ophthalmology. A Practical Guide to Disorders of the Eyes and their Management*, 2nd edn. World Scientific, Singapore.

5 Cullen AP (1981) Unmasking red eye's cause. *Rev Optom* July, pp. 44–52.

6 Ben Ezra D, Bonini S, Carreras B *et al.* (1994) Guidelines on the diagnosis and treatment of conjunctivitis. *Ocular Immunol Inflammat* **2** (suppl): S1–S55.

7 Millichamp NJ, Dziezyk J (1991) Mediators of oculr inflammation. *Prog Vet Comp Ophthalmol* **1**: 41–48.

8 Fujishima H, Takeyama M, Takeuchi T *et al.* (1997) Elevated levels of substance P in tears of patients with allergic conjunctivitis and vernal keratoconjunctivitis. *Clin Exptl Allergy* **27**: 372–378.

9 Doughty MJ (1996) Diagnostic and therapeutic pharmaceutical agents for use in contact lens practice. In: *Clinical Contact Lens Practice* (Bennett ED, Weissman BA, eds). JB Lippincott, Philadelphia, USA Chapter 9, pp. 1–38.

10 Doughty MJ (1996) Sodium cromoglycate ophthalmic solution as a pharmacy medicine for the management of mild-to-moderate, non-infectious inflammation of the conjunctiva in adults. *Ophthalmol Physiol Opt* **16** (suppl 2): S33–S38.

11 Doughty MJ (1997) A guide to ophthalmic pharmacy medicines in the United Kingdom. *Ophthal Physiol Opt* **17** (suppl 1): S2–S8.

12 Bron A, Hornby S, Tiffany J *et al.* (1997) The management of dry eyes. *Optician* **214**: 13–19.

13 Tickner J (1997) The treatment of dry eye syndrome by punctal occlusion. *Optician* **213**: 22–26.

14 Soparkar CNS, Wilhelmus KR, Koch DD *et al.* (1997) Acute and chronic conjunctivitis due to over-the-counter ophthalmic decongestants. *Arch Ophthalmol* **115**: 34–38.

15 Dostert P, Benedetti MS, Poggesi I (1997) Review of the pharmacokinetics and metabolism of reboxetine, a selective noradrenaline reuptake inhibitor. *Eur Neuropsychopharmacol* **7** (S–1): S23–S35.

16 De Boer T (1995) The effects of mirtazapine on central noradrenergic and serotonergic neurotransmission. *Int Clin Psychopharmacol* **10** (suppl 4): 19–23.

17 Doughty MJ (1999) Re-wetting, comfort, lubricant and moisturising solutions for the contact lens wearer. *Contact Lens Anterior Eye* **22**: 116-126.

18 Christensen MT, Barry JR, Turner FD (1998) Five-minute removal of soft lenses prevents most absorption of a topical ophthalmic solution. *CLAO J* **24**: 227–231.

19 Dechant KL, Goa KL (1991) Levocabastine. A review of its pharmacological properties and therapeutic potential as a topical antihistamine in allergic rhinitis and conjunctivitis. *Drugs* **41**: 202–224.

20 Horak F, Berger UE, Menapace R *et al.* (1998) Dose-dependent protection by azelastine eye drops against pollen-induced allergic conjunctivitis. *Drug Res* **48**: 379–384.

21 Discepola M, Deschenes J, Abelson M (1999) Comparison of the topical ocular antiallergic efficacy of emedastine 0.05% ophthalmic solution to ketorolac 0.5% ophthalmic solution in a clinical model of allergic conjunctivitis. *Acta Ophthalmol Scand* **77**: 43–46.

22 Ciprandi G, Buscaglia S, Cerqueti PM *et al.* (1992) Drug treatment of allergic conjunctivitis. A review of the evidence. *Drugs* **43**: 154–176.

23 Kivisto KT, Neuvonen PJ, Klotz U (1994) Inhibition of terfenadine metabolism. Pharmacokinetic and pharmacodynamic consequences. *Clin Pharmacokinet* **27**: 1–5.

# 7
# Medication-related adverse drug reactions (ADRs) – extra and intraocular muscles

Medication-related adverse drug reactions and eye muscles
Systemic medications and palpebral aperture
Systemic medications and eyeblink activity
Systemic medications and eye movement control
Systemic medications and accommodation
Systemic medications and the pupil

## Introduction

Many drugs in systemically administered medicines act on the central nervous system (CNS) and/or autonomic nervous system and can affect the muscles of the eye.[1] Such iatrogenic effects have long been recognised by medical practitioners.[2] Some adverse drug reactions (ADRs) affecting the eye muscles were reported to the College of Optometrists via the green card scheme that was in operation until the end of 1998.[3] Such induced changes can unquestionably be a cause of significant vision changes.[4]

There is a wide range of neuropharmacological mechanisms that can cause these effects (see Chapter 3). In Chapter 5 the action of these drugs on smooth muscle or muscle-like (myoepithelial) systems of secretory systems and the peripheral vasculature were considered since an understanding of these types of changes is important in the differential diagnosis of diseases of the external eye, i.e. as affecting the tear film and conjunctiva.

However, for well-understood pharmacokinetic reasons, many of these drugs will also reach the other muscular systems of the eye and exert subtle to substantial effects. These drugs can reach the eye muscles via the general systemic circulation or secretory sites within or around the eye (see Chapters 1 and 2).

## General perspectives on detecting and monitoring medication-related ADRs on eye muscles

Systemic drug interactions with the various eye muscles need to be considered for a variety of reasons. These can range from effects on coordinated eye motion and pupil reactions to manifest refractive error, and a range of terms can be applied to these iatrogenic effects on the eye and vision (Table 7.1).

As with reporting potential effects of systemic medication on lacrimation and the conjunctiva (see Chapter 5), a pharmaceutical directory is unlikely to contain many details of any effects on the eye muscles nor use specific terminology of the type readers are accustomed to using. For example, disorders of binocular vision are unlikely to be reported as diplopia; instead such non-descript terms as blurred vision or transient visual changes will be used.

---

**Table 7.1 Types of ocular neuromuscular ADRs and descriptive terms (terminology) often used**[*]

- Blurred vision
- (Temporary) vision disturbances
- Blepharospasm
- Involuntary eye (muscle) movements
- Myoclonus
- Increased/decreased palpebral aperture
- Decreased convergence/convergence insufficiency
- Reduced fusional reserves
- Paresis of extraocular muscles
- Oculogyric crisis
- Decreased spontaneous eye movement
- Nystagmus
- Jerky pursuit movements
- Diplopia
- Reduced (amplitude of) accommodation
- Accommodative insufficiency
- Pseudomyopia/refractive error changes
- Mydriasis/pupil dilation
- Miosis/pupil constriction

[*] Such a list cannot be comprehensive but is merely a guide to the wide range of terms that can be encountered for ADRs that affect eye muscle function

This is simply because the true aetiology of patient complaints is rarely investi- gated, yet, the author would argue, consideration of these aetiologies is an essential part of the diagnoses of both visual dysfunction and a wide range of other patient symptoms, even if subtle.

Similarly, a drug causing mydriasis is unlikely to have this listed as an ADR in pharmaceutical directories, yet it could clearly be a cause of enhanced light sensitivity that in itself may be causing a patient to complain of photophobia and thus also be reported as a form of visual disturbance.

Equally importantly, any listing that notes a contraindication (C/I) for the use of a medicine as 'glaucoma' should prompt practitioners to consider not only that the likely meaning of this is 'narrow-angle glaucoma', but also that these medicines could thus be expected to cause subtle changes in pupillary light reflexes, some degree of mydriasis, and often affect near vision to some extent.

Some drugs in this category not only put the eye at risk for such severe events as iatrogenic angle-closure but, if they have the appropriate pharmacological mechanisms, they could also change accommodation and binocular vision driven vergence and near-point vision. They could thus be a cause of blurred vision (depending on the patient's age, manifest refraction and the nature of any extraocular correction habitually worn).

A number of medications in this group are actually mentioned – usually under specific precautions (S/P) or possible inter- actions (INT) listings in a pharmaceutical directory – for a range of anti-glaucoma medications. Such listings both underlie the potential for drug effects on the pupil as well as there being a chance of systemic interactions. An understanding of such potential interactions should be part of the comprehensive monitoring of glaucoma patients or glaucoma suspects.

It is difficult to predict who will show eye-related neuromuscular ADRs. One important aspect of systemic medication-induced changes in eye muscle activities relates to drug biotransformation (see Chapter 1). If individuals show slower rates of biotransformation (and often also in the resultant bioelimination), then higher peak drugs levels will be realised in the circulation. If the volume of distribution (Chapter 1) is also relatively small, then pronounced neuromuscular ADRs can follow, e.g. in children or frail and underweight adults.

Differences in drug metabolism can be a result of disease or of pharmacogenetic differences between individuals. One individual may have lower levels of enzyme(s) that metabolise drugs. Alcohol is one good example, but such biotransformation interactions have been also documented for well-known drugs specifically for the eye, e.g. atropine and pilocarpine, which are metabolised by a non-specific esterase (sometimes called atropine or pilocarpine esterase).[5]

Similarly, individuals can show remarkably different rates of metabolism to many antidepressant drugs (tricyclic antidepressants, etc) and so determine the kinetics and magnitude of any ADRs.

The possibility of drug–drug or food–drug interactions as a determination of altered biotransformation should also be considered. The recent substantial attention given to metabolism of the histamine $H_1$-antagonists, terfenadine and astemizole, is one such example (see Chapter 6).

## Systemic medications and palpebral aperture

These ADRs will affect the habitual resting position of the eyelids (Figure 7.1). Such changes in the palpebral aperture could result in changes in tear film stability, especially if the palpebral aperture is wider, although such potential effects are poorly understood. It is known, however, that the involuntary closure of the eyelids, as well as voluntary and reflex closing, requires the coordinated activity of both sympathetic- and parasympathetic-controlled eyelid muscles and these are generally under the influence of mixed CNS receptors and nuclei (nerve centres) including GABA-, dopamine-, histamine- and acetylcholine-mediated synapses.[6]

A mild ptosis that is usually transient or periodic can thus develop with use of a range of CNS-active drugs;[1] such effects can generally be expected to depend on the dose of the medication and when it was taken (a chronopharmacological effect). The impact of such a ptosis can range from a heavy lid sensation, to developing

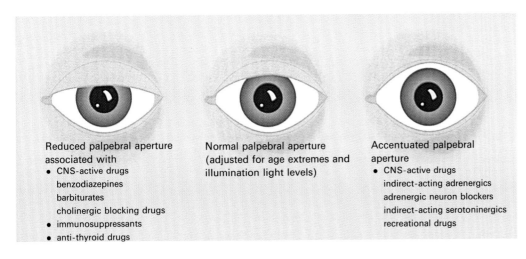

Reduced palpebral aperture associated with
- CNS-active drugs
  benzodiazepines
  barbiturates
  cholinergic blocking drugs
- immunosuppressants
- anti-thyroid drugs

Normal palpebral aperture (adjusted for age extremes and illumination light levels)

Accentuated palpebral aperture
- CNS-active drugs
  indirect-acting adrenergics
  adrenergic neuron blockers
  indirect-acting serotoninergics
  recreational drugs

**Figure 7.1**
*Changes in palpebral aperture as a consequence of use of systemic medications. The position of the upper eyelid margin with respect to the cornea and pupil should be noted.*

intolerance to rigid contact lens wear. It can also become cosmetically unacceptable to the patient.

GABA-ergic drugs are the more likely causes of a reduction in the palpebral aperture, e.g. habitual use of benzodiazepine tranquillisers/sleep aids such as nitrazepam, or high dosing with hypnotic sedatives/tranquillisers such as benzodiazepines or barbiturates.[1,7]

However, there is anecdotal evidence that certain other drugs may cause a slight ptosis that could actually be beneficial. An example would be the range of drugs for refractory arthritis which can exert a general non-specific neuromuscular blocking effect in addition to immunosuppression, e.g. hydroxychloroquine.[1] Such an effect can perhaps be used to advantage since it has been anecdotally noted that it can reduce ocular symptoms in rheumatoid arthritis patients suffering from more severe forms of dry eye.[8]

A similar perspective should be taken when patients are taking any medications that should ameliorate the signs and symptoms of eye diseases such as those associated with hyperthyroidism.

Systemic medications can also cause a slight widening (0.5 to 1 mm) of the palpebral aperture, which may be of consequence for rigid contact lens wear fitting, or in borderline cases of inadequate lid closure, and could lead to exposure keratitis (see Chapter 6). Such a 'wide-eyed' effect is part of the 'fright-and-flight' response originating at the sympathetically innervated Müller's muscle and could occur following the use of a wide range of drugs that act as CNS stimulants with direct or indirect-acting adrenergic or serotoninergic effects (see Chapter 3).

These should include those used for medicinal (e.g. ephedrine, MAO inhibitors, NaSSAs, SNRIs, NARIs) or recreational purposes (e.g. amphetamines, cocaine, etc).[1,6]

There are miscellaneous reports indicating that such a widening of the palpebral aperture could be linked to an increased blink rate (see below) but this has yet to be studied in detail. An alternative means of temporarily and substantially widening the palpebral aperture (via the levator muscle) is that which can be achieved following acute dosing (usually *im*) with the special indirect-acting cholinergic, edrophonium.[9] This can be used as part of the clinical work-up for diagnosis of myasthenia gravis.

Other indirect-acting cholinergics are unlikely to realise sufficiently high circulatory levels after oral administration to change the palpebral aperture.

## Systemic medications and eyeblink activity

A range of drugs in systemic medications have potential effects on eyeblink activity. As with the palpebral aperture, the consequences of such changes will depend on the individual patient. Notwithstanding, it can be noted that a certain level of spontaneous blink activity is considered to be essential to the maintenance of a stable preocular tear film, although there are few quantitative data to support this.[10]

When cases of tear film instability are encountered, consideration should be given to what a patient's spontaneous eyeblink activity might be, and/or whether he or she executes complete or incomplete blinks and when there is adequate eyelid closure (Figure 7.2). A range of CNS-acting drugs,[1,6] including those with potential sedative effects, might reduce spontaneous eyeblink activity and/or reduce the palpebral aperture (see below).

Equally importantly, neuroleptic or anxiolytic-associated changes in blink patterns could be responsible for disturbance of the tear film and it is important to note that there has been sporadic reporting of such changes with a range of dopaminergic agonists (which increase blink rate) and dopamine antagonists (which decrease the blink rate).[6] GABA-ergic drugs and cholinergic blocking drugs may also reduce spontaneous as well as reflex blink rates slightly.

The alcohol consumption of a patient should be considered. While the dysfunction of binocular vision following ingestion of excessive alcohol is well known,[11] the secondary consequences may easily be overlooked. For example, a social drinker

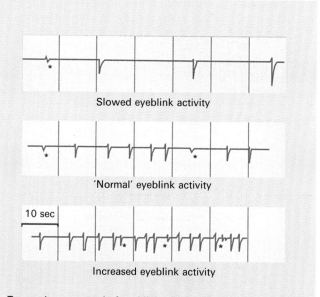

Traces show a record of eyeblink activity with the downward deflections indicating eyelid closure. It is not known whether the number or pattern of eyeblinks is important to maintain a tear film. Incomplete blinks are indicated*

**Figure 7.2**

*Changes in spontaneous eyeblink activity associated with use of systemic medications. Blink frequency can fall dramatically if sedation occurs and increase dramatically if a patient is uncomfortable or has irritated eyes, etc. Concentration on a visual task can reduce eyeblink frequency while even casual conversation can increase it significantly. Notwithstanding, from a uniform pattern of blinking (centre), medications may decrease (top) or increase (bottom) the activity.*

could well develop borderline dry-eye symptoms not only because of the potential effects of ethyl alcohol on tear film secretion (see Chapter 5), but also because of repeated periods of perturbation or even disruption of that type of eyeblink activity required to maintain a stable tear film in a particular patient.

## Systemic medications and eye movement control

A range of different types of drugs can affect the coordination of the extraocular muscles and therefore the normal positioning of the eyes and how the eyes respond to visual cues. A number of systemic drugs affect the neuromuscular system by slowing down voluntary and involuntary control of muscle function throughout the body; they may be manifest as subtle alterations in spontaneous eyeblink activity.

In susceptible individuals and at higher doses of anxiolytic medications (benzodiazepines, e.g. nitrazepam), such interactions can result in slowing of ocular saccades. In rare cases, the symptoms experienced will go beyond patients simply considering something is not quite right with their binocular vision, to them actually noting diplopia.

However, there is insufficient detail in the ADR literature to indicate whether different drugs will cause crossed or uncrossed diplopia, or produce types of asymmetric convergence or other abnormalities of (uniocular) motor control.

There is a further extension of such drug-induced changes in extraocular muscle function in that, presumably as a result of the extraordinary coupling between the sets of extraocular muscles, one or more muscle groups can become differentially affected or even temporarily 'paralysed', i.e. fail to respond to normally yoked neural stimuli and so result in a paresis of one or more extraocular muscles.

That drugs can substantially affect the extraocular muscle function is well known since a manifest nystagmus (which is often of the pendular type and develops especially at extremes of gaze) is a familiar consequence of even moderate alcohol consumption.[12] Such irregularity of extraocular muscle control reflects one aspect of the fine control of stereopsis.

A probable precursor, likely to go unnoticed with alcohol intoxication, is the

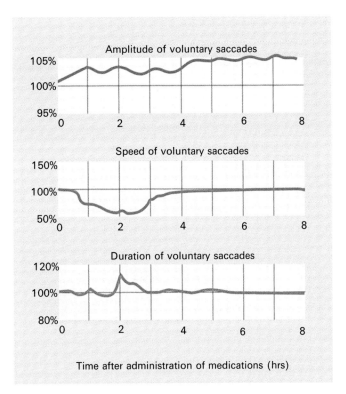

**Figure 7.3**
*Time-dependent changes in monocular pursuit eye movements following administration of CNS-active drugs.*

earlier phases of these effects that are reported as some form of blurred vision and which result from a slowing down of pursuit saccades (Figure 7.3). Such slowing of neuromuscular activity is probably the result of CNS-originating sedative effects.

This general conclusion can be applied regardless of whether the offending medicines contain benzodiazepines,[13] tricyclic antidepressants,[14] or sedating antihistamines.[15] In addition to episodic blurred vision, functions such as hand–eye coordination may be significantly impaired,[16,17] as may be any tasks requiring coordination,[18] as the slowed extraocular muscle (EOM) responses to near-point stimuli produce a form of convergence insufficiency.

Such effects are more likely to be cumulative, as a result of repeated administration of the offending medications, with fusional reserves initially being adequate to compensate for the drug-induced effect. However, as a patient tires and/or stress develops, the effects could become much more pronounced.

In rare cases, the dysfunction in eye muscle control is so substantial that there is a total loss of interocular control and one eye turns out (a type of toxic amblyopia) or upwards (an element of an oculogyric crisis) with both eyes generally showing intermittent uncontrolled movements before and after such extreme events.

A pharmaceutical directory such as *MIMS* lists such ADRs under a range of descriptions such as visual disturbances, CNS disturbances, extrapyramidal symptoms or reactions, or involuntary motor activities. The CNS receptors affected by these drugs range from those mediated by GABA (e.g. with the use of anxiolytics such as nitrazepam), dopamine (e.g. clinical use of dopaminergic blockers such as metoclopramide), or acetylcholine (e.g. the clinical use of CNS-active cholinergic blockers such as benztropine, or drugs such as tricyclic or tetracyclic antidepressants which can have significant cholinergic blocking side-effects).

None of these effects is common and it is only from contemporary medicines trials that we can even start to get some real estimates of how often these sorts of ADRs might be encountered. Despite such uncertainty, the more substantial and bizarre

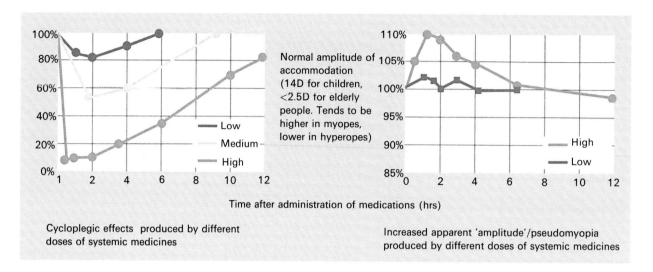

**Figure 7.4**
*Time-dependent changes in the amplitude of accommodation after the oral administration of medicines, adjusted for age-dependent differences.*

effects, such as an oculogyric crisis, are more likely to occur with drugs that have dual actions in the CNS. These substantial effects have been reported, for example, for the phenothiazine neuroleptics such as chlorpromazine used as major tranquillisers,[19] or the tricyclic antidepressant-related drug carbamazepine used for control of epilepsy;[20] both have actions on the dopaminergic and cholinergic systems (see Chapter 3).

The newer dopamine-acetylcholine gastrokinetic agents such as metoclopramide can also cause oculogyric crises,[21] to the extent that some specialists recommend that initial dosing should be in a clinic or hospital so patients can be monitored for these reactions. With newer drugs, for instance the dopaminergic/serotoninergic antagonists such as risperidone, some effects on saccades velocity have already been reported,[22] but it remains to be seen if substantial ADRs can occur.

For drugs expected to have substantial anticholinergic side-effects (e.g. the tricyclic antidepressants), significant ADRs of this type are more likely to come from overdose,[23] yet, with these drugs being used for depression, the chance of inadvertent overdosing must be considered as significant.

From slight blurring of vision, to reported diplopia, to a manifest nystagmus, the magnitude of the effects that can be observed depends not only on drug dosing but also on when the medications were taken. As a rough guide, the period 1–4

hours after administration of medications is when there is the greatest chance of clinically relevant changes occurring, especially with cumulative effects and fatigue also being considered. In a medicolegal climate, the informed patient can expect to be advised of any such difficulties with performance (even if they elect to then ignore them). Residual effects may be detected by careful evaluation of ocular convergence (i.e. AC/A ratios and similar).[24–26]

All of these extrapyramidal or vestibular effects should subside once the medication is discontinued, at which point compensatory disturbances in binocular vision may also occur. This can be especially important when the medications are being used for conditions that, in themselves, may precipitate some form of incomitancy, e.g. migraine accompanied by fluctuating eye movement control when CNS-acting antimigraine drugs are used. These might include the serotoninergic antagonists such as pergolide, or the Ca-blocker/serotoninergic, flunarizine.[27]

In other conditions, such as epilepsy, the anti-epilepsy medications may simply attenuate or otherwise alter ocular motor reactions to visual stimuli that the patient has become accustomed to, with the result that nystagmus or other more substantial and uncontrollable episodic eye movement disorders follow, e.g. after the use of CNS-active drugs for epilepsy such as carbamazepine, gabapentin or phenytoin.[28]

## Systemic medications and accommodation

A large range of drugs can cause cycloplegic effects, and a few can produce over-accommodation.

Many systemic drugs can interact with the ciliary body to relax it, while a few have the potential to increase the tone of the ciliary body (Figure 7.4). In either case, the patient may report some type of blurred vision, depending on their refractive error and habitual correction.

From an eye examination perspective, these systemic drugs most commonly produce a partial reduction in the measurable amplitude of accommodation, with or without full spectacle correction. Such an effect may be dramatic, so the patient suddenly notices blur at near due to an obvious cycloplegic effect of the systemic medications. Often, however, the effect is more subtle and first noticed 6–12 hours after medication, as the accommodation/vergence system starts to tire after being overexerted for near-point tasks to try to overcome the mild cycloplegic effects of the systemic medications.

Any assessment of refractive error and/or true spectacle needs should generally be postponed until the medication use is reduced or discontinued.

Since it is often considered that the parasympathetic innervation to the ciliary body dominates that of the sympathetic system, the first group of drugs that are likely to cause a cycloplegic effect are those with an atropine-like action. Even the systemic administration of these drugs may be enough to cause dramatic visual effects, both as a result of the cycloplegia and the substantial pupil dilation that accompanies the cycloplegia.[29,30]

Atropine-like drugs have a wide number of uses to manage ailments of the gastrointestinal and urinary tract, such as diarrhoea (e.g. hyoscine), urinary incontinence (e.g. oxybutynin) and travel sickness (e.g. hyoscine). It is important also to consider the potential cycloplegic effects of a wide range of systemic drugs that have cholinergic-blocking (atropine-like) side-effects, especially if administered at high doses. These include phenothiazine antipsychotic drugs/tranquillisers (chlorpromazine, etc),[31] standard doses of anti-arrhythmia drugs such as disopyramide,[32] and high doses of tricyclic antidepressants (trimipramine, etc).[33,34]

Drugs with indirect sympathomimetic effects should not be overlooked as some individuals can show substantial cycloplegia to sympathomimetics,[35] and it is possible that similar effects could occur when indirect adrenergics (e.g. MAO inhibitors such as phenelzine) are administered orally,[36] i.e. especially in high myopes.

There is also evidence to suggest that the opposite can occur, i.e. a CNS-mediated (alpha$_2$)/peripheral sympatholytic drug effect that would 'increase' accommodation, with the important result that convergence accommodation (CA) may then be proportionately different to CNS-driven accommodative convergence (AC), leading to an insufficiency.[37]

A few drugs are more generally recognised as causing a measurable myopic shift in manifest refractive error. Pseudomyopia is the term given to an involuntary over-accommodation that results from a drug-induced contracture of the ciliary body; this will often be accompanied by a miosis. The effect generally will be noticeable in patients with reasonable reliance on their accommodation for (near) vision. In susceptible patients with already limited fusional reserves, the miotic-driven accommodative change could be enough to drive an intermittent (exo)phoria or even some types of nystagmus.[38]

Strong cholinergic drugs used as micturating agents in cases of urinary retention (e.g. oral bethanechol) would be expected to exert a parasympathetic effect on the ciliary body/accommodation of younger individuals; blurred vision is thus a listed ADR. Similarly, morphine and morphine-like drugs can cause pseudomyopia as well as pupil miosis (see later).

What needs to be noted also is that the pseudomyopia could be accompanied by pupillary block and secondary angle-closure.[39,40] The same risk could be considered to apply to other drugs causing pseudomyopia, although the number of cases of serious complications is probably very small.

Overall, the mechanisms underlying the pseudomyopia caused by these other drugs is less clear, although they would appear to involve the relative fluid balance of the ciliary body, i.e. these agents change this balance with respect to the surrounding tissues and the vasculature.

Alternatively, a myopic shift can occur that does not directly involve the muscle but the rest of the ciliary body. Such changes in the fluid balance of the ciliary body can be enough indirectly to alter the position of the muscles such that it seems as if the muscle contracted, i.e. a forward movement of the lens associated with oedema of the ciliary body. The latter effects are short lived but can be enough to be troublesome to a patient. In all cases, the effects are likely to be accompanied by a shallowing of the anterior chamber.

Management simply includes noting the effects and, in most cases, rescheduling any spectacle corrections to a time when the drug therapy has been reduced or discontinued. These drugs include those that have obvious effects on fluid secretion such as the histamine H$_2$-blocking drugs (e.g. cimetidine used as antigastric ulcer drugs), or potent diuretics (e.g. carbonic anhydrase inhibitors such as acetazolamide).[41]

Less clear is why some antibiotics or anti-infectives (e.g. tetracyclines and sulphonamides[42]) can cause measurable pseudomyopia; the refractive changes are accompanied by a marked shallowing of the anterior chamber which suggests that there is significant forward movement of the crystalline lens.

## Systemic medications and the pupil

As with drugs with potential cycloplegic effects, there are many systemic medications capable of dilating the pupil, and a few that can close the pupil, as well as causing a myopic shift (Figure 7.5).

In the majority of cases, the resultant effects will be largely inconsequential, yet a comprehensive knowledge and understanding of drugs that fall into this group can be important as part of general testing of pupil function and ocular health examinations (through routine pupillary dilation[43,44]), as well as being an essential part of the selection of some antiglaucoma drugs (see Chapter 10).[45]

The pupil, and its responsivity to light and near-point stimuli, is extraordinarily sensitive to both sympathetic and parasympatholytic drugs. A slight but nonetheless clinically significant increase in pupil size can occur and/or there is simply a slowing of the light and near-point responses of the pupil. It can be expected that the more the resting state of the pupil is affected, the more likely it is that the reactions to light stimuli will be slowed or even absent.

It is important to distinguish such effects from general sedation, which can cause a gradual slowing of pupil responses and even slight miosis.[46] If the effect is generally symmetrical, then patients may experience enhanced light sensitivity (photophobia) as a first symptom, followed by blur, especially if the accommodation and convergence are affected as well (see above).

It might be argued that the effects generally would be expected to be symmetrical (i.e. no Marcus Gunn phenomenon evident), although common conditions such as migraine can produce substantial anisocoria and asymmetry in pupil sensitivity to drugs.[5,27] In rare circumstances, the consequences may not only be asymmetrical but constitute an ocular emergency when angle-closure develops, with the patient presenting with only one eye substantially affected (see below).

For either bilateral or uniocular effects, any mydriasis associated with systemic medication use is unlikely to be more than 1 mm. However, when substantial doses of the systemic medications are taken in some individuals, there is always a chance for a much more substantial dilation or the fixing of the pupil in the mid-dilated position. Since the changes in the pupil diameter can generally be expected to follow a predictable time course (pharmacokinetics, see Chapter 2), noting the time of medication administration is an essential part of evaluating such patients.

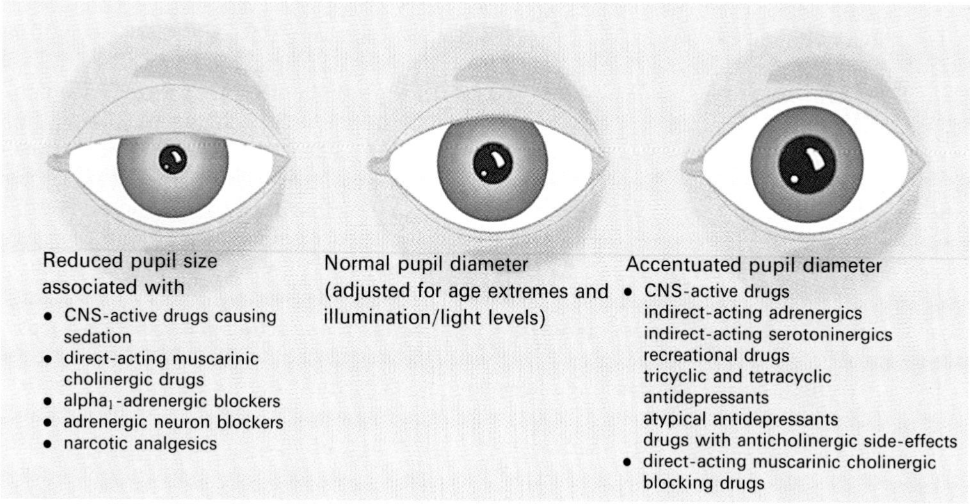

**Reduced pupil size associated with**
- CNS-active drugs causing sedation
- direct-acting muscarinic cholinergic drugs
- alpha₁-adrenergic blockers
- adrenergic neuron blockers
- narcotic analgesics

**Normal pupil diameter** (adjusted for age extremes and illumination/light levels)

**Accentuated pupil diameter**
- CNS-active drugs
  indirect-acting adrenergics
  indirect-acting serotoninergics
  recreational drugs
  tricyclic and tetracyclic antidepressants
  atypical antidepressants
  drugs with anticholinergic side-effects
- direct-acting muscarinic cholinergic blocking drugs

**Figure 7.5**

*Changes in resting pupil size as a consequence of use of systemic medications. The relative size of the pupil with respect to the corneal limbus should be noted.*

The primary reason for this is that even a very slight pupil effect (which would indicate that enough drug was entering the eye from the systemic circulation) could translate to a substantial effect when illumination levels are lower, at the end of the day for example.[47]

This risk of angle-closure in susceptible eyes (e.g. those with narrow anterior chamber angles[43,44]) is real and the reason why there are so many small notes in the pharmaceutical directories listing 'glaucoma' as a C/I or where 'glaucoma' is listed under S/P notes. It is a useful exercise to use a highlighter to mark all these notes in the directory so the information is then included in a patient's records.

A case can be made that any systemic medication that dilates the pupil could pose a risk for angle-closure in susceptible patients, yet it should also be considered whether all such drugs pose the same risks. Since the angle-closure is perhaps more likely to develop via iris seclusion (pupillary block), it can be argued that if the pupil retains some light reactivity, then the risk of angle-closure should be less. Such ideas cannot be used to define management strategies, but should temper risk assessments.

Notwithstanding, the management of all such patients should include providing screening for narrow anterior chamber angles, or shallow anterior chamber angles, with the view to identifying any patients at risk and/or with a history of intermittent angle-closure. Timely referral of

patients back to the person who prescribed the medications is important when at-risk or problem cases are encountered.

The provision of patient counselling is appropriate for use of certain OTC (P medicines) products in relation to the anterior chamber angle and the pupil (see Chapter 6).[48]

As indicated above, there are a large number of notes in the pharmaceutical directory indicating that the risk of angle-closure should be considered. Atropine-like drugs can dilate the pupil, and a number of drugs of this type are used for alimentary tract ailments associated with stomach cramps, irregular bowel movements, diarrhoea, motion sickness, etc, including the modern-day ailment of irritable bowel syndrome (IBS). These include drugs such as hyoscine, dicyclomine, and propantheline. Some drugs in this class can also occasionally be used to control urinary incontinence, e.g. oxybutynin.

There are other very special uses of cholinergic-blocking drugs, e.g. ipratropium used in aerosols as an anti-asthma drug or in sprays as an antirhinorrhoea drug. With such delivery modes, it is entirely possible that some of the drug is inadvertently delivered to the eye via the conjunctival route as opposed to the nasal–bronchial route. In addition, certain antiarrhythmia agents such as disopyramide, neuroleptics (for instance the phenothiazines), and presumably most (if not all) of

the tricyclic and tetracyclic antidepressants and the atypical antipsychotics (e.g. clozapine) also have cholinergic-blocking properties. Even if not immediately recognised as having atropine-like or anticholinergic effects, the use of these types of drug can still cause unexpected angle-closure.[27,49,50] All these drugs have anticholinergic ADRs and the potential to dilate the pupil. Thus their directory listings carry C/I or S/P notes relating to (angle-closure) glaucoma.

Overall, it is the enormous range of second-generation tricyclic and tetracyclic drugs that are today still perhaps the most likely to precipitate angle-closure,[51] yet there are a number of other categories of drugs that could equally precipitate such crises because of their widespread use. Certain antihistamines used for substantial allergies, as sleep aids or for nausea have the potential for substantial anticholinergic side-effects. For instance, promazine, diphenhydramine, and bromo- or chlorpheniramine have all been reported to produce mydriasis.[1]

Perhaps the greatest potential for unexpected cases of angle-closure glaucoma comes from the expanding use of drugs with autonomic mechanisms of action yet for which there is, at the time of writing, only limited evidence for effects on the pupil.

Indirect adrenergics such as the traditional MAO inhibitors (e.g. phenelzine) rarely precipitate angle-closure. The listings for use of this group of drugs and/or use of other sympathomimetics (e.g. ephedrine and phenylephrine) include C/I and S/P for glaucoma. It should not be overlooked, however, that there are now reversible (e.g. RIMAs, moclobemide) and selective (e.g. selegiline) inhibitors of monoamine oxidase. In addition, with the rapidly expanding range of other indirect-acting adrenergic types, these must be recognised as potential causes of unwanted pupillary dilation and thus a risk of angle-closure,[43] e.g. new drugs such as reboxetine, a noradrenaline-reuptake inhibitor.[52]

As a matter of contingency, the widely prescribed indirect-acting serotoninergic antidepressants (the SSRIs such as fluoxetine, POM Prozac) should also be listed with the other antidepressants for due consideration of ocular safety. There are two reasons for this. First, even though co-administration of SSRIs with or shortly following other adrenergic antidepressants is not generally recommended, it is nonetheless likely that patients prescribed SSRIs could earlier have been taking indirect adrenergics, tricyclics or tetracyclics and it would be unwise to assume that the effects of SSRIs can be completely separated from the indirect adrenergics.

Secondly, while it could be argued that traditional pharmacological analysis of the pupil does not include a serotoninergic mechanism, this is simply because it has not been studied in any detail, and it is important to note that even SSRIs (e.g. paroxetine) can apparently exert some systemic parasympatholytic/adrenergic effects (causing blurred vision) including pupil dilation and angle-closure.[53]

As a final note on pupil-dilating drugs, attention should be given to those that might often be ignored, e.g. special amphetamine-like drugs such as methylphenidate (POM Ritalin). The recreational use of a range of serotoninergic drugs including LSD and amphetamines can produce similar adrenergic effects for a variety of reasons.[1,54]

The overuse or deliberate abuse of direct-acting adrenergics as nasal decongestants, albeit in dilute solutions, could still precipitate angle-closure in a susceptible individual and these products also carry a S/P note about 'glaucoma', e.g. xylometazoline or oxymetazoline.[48]

In terms of evaluation (by providing an eye examination for a GP or even on referral from a pharmacist), monitoring or providing advice on such patients, similar guidelines to those used to assess eyes before deliberate pupil dilation[43] should be followed, i.e. those medications capable of causing mydriasis should be contraindicated in a patient with anterior chamber angles considered at risk for closure.

This author, despite asking, is not aware of any formal guidelines concerning the concurrent use of these systemic medications in patients with anterior-chamber IOLs or with diseases that carry a risk of crystalline lens subluxation. Caution is surely appropriate in such patients, which may prompt a practitioner to seek advice and request an eye examination.

Miosis, of course, is a smaller-than-usual pupil size but this is much harder to gauge compared with mydriasis. Substantial age- and disease-dependent (e.g. advanced diabetes mellitus) miosis can develop; a smaller resting pupil can make a drug-induced miosis more difficult to detect. Perhaps a better way of detecting whether a medication-related miosis is present is to assess the opposite, i.e. whether a pupil will dilate when the light levels are lowered.

In younger individuals, an accompanying pseudomyopia (see above) may also be an easier way to detect whether a systemic medication is causing miosis.

The consequences of a medication-induced miosis are not certain as only a handful of these drugs are actually used, but some do carry a note about cholinergic side-effects and/or list a cholinergic ocular side-effect (e.g. lacrimation for oral pilocarpine, blurred vision for oral bethanechol). Management will thus generally not need to be taken beyond noting the occurrence of the adverse reaction, unless, of course, a patient's vision is actually compromised.

As an example, in an elderly patient already suffering senile miosis, further constriction of the pupil following medication with indirect-acting cholinergics such as bethanechol (for urinary retention) or donepezil (for Alzheimer's disease) could precipitate 'blurred vision' (the term used in the pharmaceutical directories) associated with miosis,[55] or, as is perhaps more likely, 'poor vision' due to inadequate retinal illumination.

The pupils of such patients may also be more difficult to dilate with tropicamide, not only because they are smaller but because the tropicamide will have to counteract the effects of the parasympathetic drug(s) on the iris sphincter as well.

There are more substantial pupillary constriction effects that can occur, but which are less likely to be a cause of concern to patients because of the circumstances under which the medications are being given. Miosis, with loss of light and near-point reflexes,[56,57] can be a noticeable characteristic following administration of opioid narcotics to accident victims since these drugs can all elicit substantial indirect parasympathetic effects.

Other morphine-related drugs (e.g. buprenorphine or pethidine) are used for the same reasons, or as postoperative analgesics, and similar reactions may develop if these are used as substances of abuse or for management of addicts (e.g. CD Methadone). For such patients, the miosis can be expected to be rapid in onset (i.e. less than 30 minutes) and persist until withdrawal from the narcotic starts 12–24 hours later; with repeated dosing, the pupil may stay slightly miotic with loss of light sensitivity.

As noted above, a general sedation or a loss of hyperexcitability (anxiety) following use of some antidepressant medicines can cause a slight miosis with sustained therapy.[58] It is unfortunate that there is apparently no way to predict how a patient will respond to antidepressants, and thus gauge whether they are more at risk of pupil dilation or constriction.

Just as pupil dilation can have a sympathetic or parasympatholytic aetiology, the opposite duality of mechanisms applies to miosis. As with newer medicines that could potentially cause pupil dilation, it is uncertain whether systemic alpha$_1$-adrenergic blockers will cause miosis. Some of these are widely used for hypertension (e.g. oral prazosin), while other are less widely used (e.g. the newer selective oral alpha$_1$-blockers such as indoramin used for urine retention in cases of prostate hypertrophy).

Special attention might, however, again be given to those elderly patients already with senile miosis where a further effect could be substantial in terms of their vision and lifestyle needs.

## Conclusions

In this chapter, the large number of ways in which systemic medications can affect the neuromuscular systems of the eye have been addressed. The goal of this chapter is not to try to make a case that iatrogenic changes in eye muscular function are commonplace, but to develop an approach to eye health care that includes these issues rather than ignoring them. Many of these drugs that can change eye muscle function have their origins of action in the CNS,[59] which means that the management of these patients requires special attention.

## References

1 Lubeck MJ (1971) Effects of drugs on ocular muscles. *Int Ophthalmol Clin* **11**: 35–61.

2 Cant JS (1969) Iatrogenic eye disease. *Practitioner* **202**: 787–795.

3 Edgar DF, Gilmartin B (1997) Ocular adverse reactions to systemic medication. *Ophthal Physiol Opt* **17** (suppl 2): S1–S7.

4 Koetting JF (1975) Ocular and visual side effects of drugs – a reconsideration. *J Am Pharm Assoc* **NS15**: 558–567, 596–600.

5 Doughty MJ, Lyle WM (1992). Ocular pharmacogenetics. In: *Genetics for Primary Eye Care Practitioners* (Fatt HV, Griffin JR, Lyle WM, eds). Butterworth-Heinemann, Toronto, Canada, pp. 179–193.

6 Karson CN (1988) Physiology of normal and abnormal blinking. *Adv Neurol* **49**: 25–37.

7 Tanaka M, Isozaki H, Inanaga K (1977) Effects of ID-540 on averaged photopalpebral reflex in man. *Japan J Pharmacol* **27**: 517–522.

8 Charleux J (1967) Traitement de la maladie de Gougerot-Sjogren. Note therapeutique a propos de deux cas. *Bull Soc Ophtalmol Fr* **67**: 339–341.

9 Oh SJ, Cho HK (1990) Endrophonium responsiveness not necessarily diagnostic of myasthenia gravis. *Muscle Nerve* **13**: 187–191.

10 Zaman ML, Doughty MJ, Button NF (1998) The exposed ocular surface and its relationship to spontaneous eyeblink rate in elderly Caucasians. *Exp Eye Res* **67**: 681–686.

11 Wegner AJ, Fahle M (1999) Alcohol and visual performance. *Progr Neuropsychopharmacol Biol Psychiat* **23**: 465–482.

12 Seedorf HH (1956) Effects of alcohol on the motor fusion reserves and stereopsis as well as on the tendency to nystagmus. *Acta Ophthalmol* **34**: 273–280.

13 Bittencort PRM, Wade P, Smith AT *et al.* (1981) The relationship between peak velocity of accadic eye movements and serum benzodiazepine concentration. *Br J Clin Pharmacol* **12**: 523–533.

14 Martin P, Meienberg O, Schmid-Burgk W *et al.* (1993) Saccadic eye movements as a quantitative measure of the sedative effect of drugs. *Neuro-Ophthalmol* **13**: 5–12.

15 Hopfenbeck JR, Cowley DS, Radant A *et al.* (1995) Effects of diphenhydramine on human eye movements. *Psychopharmacology* **118**: 280–286.

16 Large ATW, Wayte G, Turner P (1971) Promethazine on hand–eye co-ordination and visual function. *J Pharm Pharmacol* **23**: 134–135.

17 Austen DP, Gilmartin BA (1971) The effect of chlordiazepoxide on visual field, extraocular muscle balance, colour matching ability and hand–eye co-ordination in man. *Br J Physiol Opt* **26**: 161–165.

18 Fine BJ, Kobrick JL, Lieberman HR *et al.* (1994) Effects of caffeine or diphenhydramine on visual vigilance. *Psychopharmacology* **114**: 233–238.

19 Gorman M, Barkley GL (1995) Oculogyric crisis induced by carbamazepine. *Epilepsia* **36**: 1158–1160.

20 Skorin L, Onofrey BE, DeWitt JD (1987) Phenothiazine-induced oculogyric crisis. *J Am Optom Assoc* **58**: 316–318.

21 Edwards M, Koo MWL, Tse RK-K (1989) Oculogyric crisis after metoclopramide therapy. *Optom Vis Sci* **66**: 179–180.

22 Sweeney JA, Bauer KS, Keshavan MS *et al.* (1997) Adverse effects of risperidone on eye movement activity: a comparison of risperidone and haloperidol in antipsychotic-naive schizophrenic patients. *Neuropsychopharmacology* **16**: 217–228.

23 Vandel P, Bonin B, Leveque E *et al.* (1997) Tricyclic antidepressant-induced extrapyramidal side effects. *Eur Neuropsychopharmacol* **7**: 207–212.

24 Cohen MM, Alpern M (1969) Vergence and accommodation. VI. The influence of ethanol on the AC-A ratio. *Arch Ophthalmol* **81**: 518–525.

25 Hogan RE, Gilmartin B (1985) The relationship between tonic vergence and oculomotor stress induced by ethanol. *Ophthal Physiol Opt* **5**: 43–51.

26 Zhai H, Goss DA, Hammond RW (1993) The effect of caffeine on the accommodative response/accommoda-

tive stimulus function and on the response AC/A ratio. *Curr Eye Res* **12**: 489–499.

27 Doughty MJ, Lyle WM (1995) Medications used to prevent migraine headaches and their potential ocular adverse effects. *Optom Vis Sci* **72**: 879–891.

28 De Cort PLM, Gielen G, Tijssen CC *et al.* (1990) The influence of antiepileptic drugs on eye movements. *Neuro-Ophthalmol* **10**: 59–68.

29 Kay CD, Morrison JD (1987) The effects of a single intramuscular injection of atropine sulphate on visual performance in man. *Human Toxicol* **6**: 165–172.

30 Parrott AC (1986) Transdermal scopolamine: effects of single and repeated patches upon aspects of vision. *Human Pyschopharmacol* **1**: 109–115.

31 Isayama Y, Yazuko Y (1967) Accommodation paresis and glaucomatic manifestations due to excessive administration of tranquilizer (phenothiazine derivatives) [in Japanese]. *Rinsho Ganka* **21**: 635–638.

32 Frucht J, Freimann I, Merin S (1984) Ocular side effects of disopyramide. *Br J Ophthalmol* **68**: 890–891.

33 Von Knorring L (1981) Changes in saliva secretion and accommodation with short term administration of imipramine and zimelidine in healthy volunteers. *Int Psychopsychiat* **16**: 69–78.

34 Santry J (1990) Medication induces accommodative infacility. *Rev Optom* **127**: 106.

35 Gimpel G, Doughty MJ, Lyle WM (1994) Large sample study of the effects of phenylephrine 2.5% eyedrops on the amplitude of accommodation in man. *Ophthal Physiol Opt* **14**: 123–128.

36 Nouri A, Cuendet JF (1971) Atteintes oculaires au cours des traitements aux thymoleptiques. *Schweiz Med Wschr* **101**: 1178–1180.

37 Tassinari J (1989) Methyldopa-related convergence insufficiency. *J Am Optom Assoc* **60**: 311–314.

38 Fish DJ, Rosen SM (1990) Epidural opioids as a cause of vertical nystagmus. *Anesthesiology* **73**: 785–786.

39 Fan JT, Johnson DH, Burk RR (1993) Transient myopia, angle-closure glaucoma, and choroidal detachment after oral acetazolamide (letter). *Am J Ophthalmol* **115**: 813–814.

40 Awan AJ, Humayun M (1984) Drug induced myopia and angle closure glaucoma in drug addiction. *Pakistan J Ophthalmol* **1**: 25–28.

41 Gallin MA, Baras I, Zweifach P (1962) Diamox-induced myopia. *Am J Ophthalmol* **54**: 237–240.

42 Grinbaum A, Ashkenazi I, Gutman I *et al.* (1993) Suggested mechanism for acute transient myopia after sulfonamide. *Ann Ophthalmol* **25**: 224–226.

43 Doughty MJ (1997) Pupillary dilation. The standard for delivery of primary eye care. Part 1. *Optometry Today* Nov 14, pp. 27–31.

44 Doughty MJ (1997) Pupillary dilation. The standard for delivery of primary eye care. Part 2. *Optometry Today* Dec 12, pp. 24–28.

45 Fingeret M (1998) Glaucoma medications, glaucoma therapy and the evolving paradigm. *J Am Optom Assoc* **69**: 115–121.

46 Kotzan JA (1978) Effect of diazepam on cognition via pupillometry. *J Pharmaceut Sci* **67**: 956–968.

47 Clark CV, Mapstone R (1986) Diurnal variation in onset of acute closed angle glaucoma. *Br Med J* **292**: 1106.

48 Doughty MJ (1997) A guide to ophthalmic pharmacy medicines in the United Kingdom. *Ophthal Physiol Opt* **17** (suppl 1): S2–S8.

49 Shah P, Dhurjon L, Metcalf T *et al.* (1992) Acute angle closure glaucoma associated with nebulised ipratropium bromide and salbutamol. *Br Med J* **304**: 40–41.

50 Trope GE, Hind VMD (1978) Closed-angle glaucoma in patient on disopyramide. *Lancet* **i**: 329.

51 Ritch R, Krupin T, Henry C *et al.* (1994) Oral impiramine and acute angle closure glaucoma. *Arch Ophthalmol* **112**: 67–68.

52 Theofilopoulos N, McDade G, Szabadi E *et al.* (1995) Effects of reboxetine and desipramine on the kinetics of the pupillary light reflex. *Br J Clin Pharmacol* **39**: 251–255.

53 Eke T, Bates AK (1997) Acute angle closure glaucoma associated with paroxetine. *Br Med J* **314**: 1387.

54 Freeman H (1958) Pupil dilation in normal and schizophrenic subjects following lysergic acid diethylamide ingestion. *Arch Neurol Psychiat* **79**: 341–344.

55 Almog S, Winkler E, Amitai Y *et al.* (1991) Acute pyridostigmine overdose: a report of nine cases. *Isr J Med Sci* **27**: 659–663.

56 Tress KH, El-Sobky AA, Aherne W, Piall E (1978) Degree of tolerance and the relationship between morphine concentration and pupil diameter following intravenous heroin in man. *Br J Clin Pharmacol* **5**: 299–303.

57 Miller CD, Asbury AJ, Brown JH (1990) Pupillary effects of alfentanil and morphine. *Br J Anaesthesia* **65**: 415–417.

58 Shur E, Checkley S, Delgado I (1993) Failure of mianserin to affect autonomic function in the pupils of depressed patients. *Acta Psychiat Scand* **67**: 50–55.

59 Doughty MJ (1999) The ocular side effects of CNS-acting drugs. *Optician* **218**: 17–26.

# 8
# Anti-infective drugs for ophthalmic use in primary eye care

Overview of goals of ocular anti-infective therapy
Mechanisms of action of general anti-infective drugs
Mechanisms of action of specific antibacterial drugs
Mechanisms of action of antiviral drugs for external eye disease
Mechanisms of action of oral antibiotics for eye disease
Clinical strategies in anti-infective therapies
Pharmaceutical availability and use
Adverse reactions to anti-infective therapies for external eye infections

## Introduction

The use of drugs with antimicrobial actions is generally indicated whenever a patient presents with the signs and symptoms of an infection affecting the external eye, or is considered at significant risk for development of an infection. Their use follows well-established principles and guidelines.[1–5]

The first strategy is one of treatment of an infection; the latter one of prophylactic treatment against infection. Both options play an important part of the management of infections of the external eye since the effective management of at-risk patients can, for example, prevent the occurrence of severe infections secondary to recurrent minor infections.

Different types of microorganisms can establish themselves on or within the tissues of the external eye, but only some of these can reasonably be considered within the realm of primary eye care. The management of ocular infections at this level should be considered as the provision of that type of diagnosis, treatment and management of a patient's eye condition that is uncomplicated, i.e. is likely to follow a predictable course that can be monitored in a systematic fashion using the equipment commonly in place in optometric practice (yet which is unlikely to be present in a general medical practice).

The overall goals of management of ocular infections at the primary care level are to prevent the further development of an infection, and to reduce the colonisation of the external eye by the offending microorganism(s) to a minimal level as quickly as reasonably possible. Such a strategy can only be realised with an understanding of the mechanisms of action of the anti-infective drugs appropriate for the conditions diagnosed at first presentation, the appropriate selection of pharmaceuticals and their use, and a commitment to the provision of follow-up care to ensure that the selected treatment options are indeed achieving the desired effect.

There is a range of terms used for the treatment of infections of the external eye and these relate to the classification of the drugs. Some drugs are true antibiotics in that they have been isolated from organisms and are known to exert adverse effects upon other microorganisms. Other drugs, while still exerting clinically useful antimicrobial actions, are partly or completely synthetic and are thus not true antibiotics. They would more appropriately be called antimicrobial drugs. However, since the clinical use of both types of drugs is to combat (or prevent) an infection, the general term anti-infective drugs is also useful.

Anti-infective drugs are often referred to in terms of whether they will simply slow down the replication rate of microorganisms (e.g. bacteria) or whether they will actually kill the cells, i.e. whether the drug(s) can be considered as bacteriostatic or bactericidal in their action. This point is rather mute from a clinical perspective since even if a drug is classified as bactericidal, it cannot achieve these effects unless a reasonably high concentration is achieved in the pertinent ocular tissue.

From this perspective, a so-called bacteriostatic drug may well be able substantially to attenuate a bacterial infection of the external eye simply because it was effectively delivered to the affected site, i.e. the pharmacokinetics of the drug dictate efficacy, not simply the mechanism of action of an ocular infective drug. Some drugs (e.g. the aminoglycoside antibiotics) can be bacteriostatic at lower concentrations but bactericidal at higher concentrations. For aminoglycosides, the mechanism by which the two effects are achieved is slightly different, but in other cases the killing effect is merely the result of a gross toxic effect unrelated to the actual specific mechanism by which a particular anti-infective drug is classified.

The drug concentrations required to achieve these '-static' or '-cidal' effects can be reported in various ways. From a simple microbiological perspective, a concentration (usually in µg/ml) of an anti-infective drug can be found that will have a specified effect on a population of microorganisms.[6–8] Perhaps one of the widest used is the MIC, or minimum inhibitory concentration. This will commonly be a concentration of drug that just affects the population of microorganisms, e.g. slows the rate of replication.

This can be ascertained fairly easily for bacteria using simple plating and culture techniques. Diluted suspensions of bacteria (e.g. as obtained from the surface of the eye) are carefully applied to the surface of a semi-solid nutritional support (e.g. agar with blood); after such an inoculation, the bacteria will replicate and spread out from the site of initial contact with the agar surface and will do so at a predictable rate unless there are, for example, antibacterial drugs present.

By comparing the relative growth of colonies of bacteria across plates containing different concentrations of antibacterial drug, an MIC can be estimated.

MIC can also be estimated by an inverse method in which the entire surface of the agar plate is smeared with a dilute suspension of bacteria. The bacteria should uniformly replicate across the entire plate and so generally increase in density unless, for example, an antibacterial drug is also applied to a portion of the surface of the agar plate. If a small disc of paper impregnated with antibacterial drug is placed on the surface of the plate, the drug can be expected to diffuse out of the filter disc and across the surface of the plate.

If the action of the drug is bacteriostatic, then the density of bacteria around the disc will be somewhat less than in areas well away from the drug-impregnated disc. If the drug is unambiguously bactericidal,

then a bacteria-free zone will be created around the drug-impregnated filter disc. A partial (bacteriostatic) or complete (bactericidal) result can be obtained using either method and both can provide an indication of whether the tested bacteria are susceptible to a certain drug. By using different concentrations of drug solutions, that which produces a bacteriostatic or bactericidal effect can be estimated.

A more refined and reliable method is to culture the bacteria in a liquid medium and actually count the number of living cells or surviving cells so that what are called 'kill curves' can be generated.[6,7] Generally these will be an assessment of the number of bacteria, for example, remaining in a solution after a 24-hour exposure to the drug. From such curves, reliable estimates of that concentration required for a 90% (e.g. $MIC_{90}$) or 50% (e.g. $MIC_{50}$) kill with a 24-hour (or other time period) exposure can be generated.

It is important to note that since many infections involve the ocular surfaces and are not really invading the ocular tissue, the concentrations of antibiotics that are often important are those that can be in the tear film over a period of 5–10 minutes after administration of eye drops or ointment.[8] Unfortunately, few such values are actually available.

For some drugs, these effective concentrations are not presented in simple gravimetric terms (i.e. µg/ml or % w/v (weight/volume), but as (International) Units (abbreviated as 'U'), e.g. 10 000 U/ml for polymyxin B and 3500 U/ml for neomycin. They measure the activity of the extracted preparation which may vary slightly from batch to batch, although a known quantity (e.g. 1 mg) of the extracted material would be expected to contain a predictable activity (e.g. 10 000 U polymyxin B/mg solid). There are agreed protocols for exactly how these relative activity measures should be done.

It should be noted that antibiotics can be extracted and purified in different ways and, as a result, different compounds can be prepared which have a different molecular weight. As a result, the molar concentrations of the compounds can differ slightly for solutions prepared on a simple w/v basis. Therefore, in some cases, antibiotic concentrations are specifically presented with respect to the base concentration, e.g. a gentamicin product is stated to contain an amount that is

equivalent to 0.3% w/v (i.e. 0.3 g/100 ml) or 3 mg/ml of the base.

## Mechanisms of action of general anti-infective drugs

A number of drugs are available that, when used appropriately, can exert general anti-infective actions for mild-to-moderate conditions affecting the external eye. These drugs were introduced into clinical use many years ago and, as a result, large-scale clinical trials are unlikely to be found in the literature. However, there is little evidence to indicate that these drugs, when appropriately used, will not be effective in the management of styes or many other infections (with inflammation) of the eyelash follicles, eyelash glands, meibomian glands or the conjunctival surface.

### Propamidine isethionate or dibromopropamidine isethionate

The mechanism of action of these diamidines includes blocking the uptake of DNA precursor molecules such as purines (Figure 8.1), but other effects include non-specific slowing of DNA synthesis.[9,10] These drugs are thus generally bacteriostatic at low concentrations and bactericidal at high concentrations.[10] The MIC for propamidine is around 10 µg/ml for common Gram-negative bacteria, but at least 20 times higher for many Gram-negative bacteria. Dibromopropamide is five times more potent.[10] Detailed pharmacokinetics for propamidine eyedrops or ointment do not appear to be available.

These drugs have general anti-infective actions and were reported to show good efficacy against both common and less prevalent types of bacterial conjunctivitis. By default, these drugs have also proven efficacious against styes and generalised blepharitis, both of which conditions can often be attributed to Gram-positive organisms such as *Staphylococcus* spp and some *Streptococcus* spp.[11,12]

Anecdotally, it appears to be accepted that the efficacy of these drugs is largely unaffected by pus or general mucopurulent discharge, with the caveat that these drugs are not meant for general treatment of severe or chronic bacterial infections of the external eye. Since the bacteriostatic activity of propamidine is pH-sensitive, when tear pH is lowered in mild infection,[13] its efficacy may vary somewhat.

**Figure 8.1**
*Antibacterial action of diamidines, such as propamidine, is the result of blocking uptake of DNA precursors into the cells.*

## Polymyxin B

Polymyxin B is a heptapeptide antibiotic which is able to insert itself into the cytoplasmic membrane of bacteria, especially Gram-negative bacteria, and perturbs or destroys the permeability control normally exerted by these membranes.[14,15] These bacterial cell membranes should not be confused with the cell wall of bacteria. This is the attribute that is used as the basis for classifying bacteria into Gram-positive (i.e. having a substantial cell wall) or Gram-negative (i.e. having a much lesser, or all-but-non-existent cell wall).

The relative sensitivity of different bacteria to polymyxin B is, in part, determined by the particular phospholipids present in their cell membranes; the fatty acid chain attached to the heptapeptide ring of polymyxin B shows different degrees of insertion into membranes according to the phospholipid side chains. With the polypeptide insertion and subsequent 'permeabilisation' of the cell membrane, the bacteria lose control of regulation of internal solutes (Figure 8.2) such that polymyxin B can be bacteriostatic at low concentrations and bactericidal at high concentrations. At high levels, polymyxin B can also perturb the outer membrane that is present in some Gram-negative bacteria.

The MIC for Gram-negative bacteria is generally $\leq 2$ μg/ml (i.e. *c* 20 U). The rate of drug penetration through the cornea for these types of polypeptides is poor, but since the primary use for polymyxin is for superficial infections, this is not important. Polymyxin B has, however, a proven efficacy against a wide range of common negative and even some Gram-positive organisms that could affect the conjunctiva and cornea.[16]

For ocular infections, polymyxin B or related antibiotics are rarely used on their own, although they have been demonstrated to have a remarkable efficacy when intensively used, even for severe ulcers.[17] In such cases, therapeutic levels are expected in the cornea tissues simply because the epithelial barrier would be lost when an ulcer is present.

## Gramicidin

Gramicidin is usually a mixture of polypeptides that exerts similar effects to polymyxin B in that it permeabilises bacterial cytoplasmic membranes.[18,19] However, the means by which this is achieved is much more selective and involves only certain ions, especially $Na^+$. The antibiotic chains form pores in the bacterial cytoplasmic membrane such that ions will very rapidly cross from one side of the membrane to the other and thus equilibrate the ionic concentrations (Figure 8.3). Without these ion gradients, especially $Na^+$ and $H^+$, the

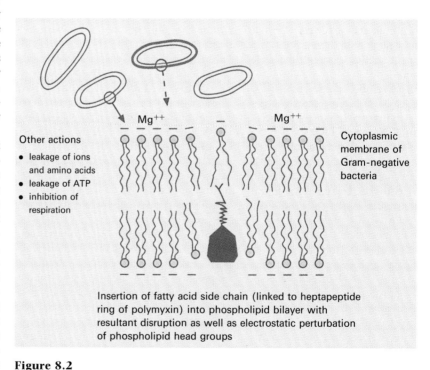

**Figure 8.2**
*Antibacterial action of polymyxin B is the result of it inserting itself into and perturbing the bacterial cytoplasmic membrane.*

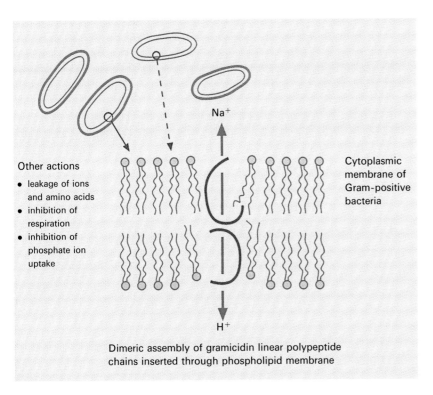

**Figure 8.3**
*Antibacterial action of gramicidin is a result of it inserting itself through the bacterial cytoplasmic membrane and making it very permeable to ions.*

Within the figure:

Na$^+$

Other actions
- leakage of ions and amino acids
- inhibition of respiration
- inhibition of phosphate ion uptake

Cytoplasmic membrane of Gram-positive bacteria

H$^+$

Dimeric assembly of gramicidin linear polypeptide chains inserted through phospholipid membrane

bacterial mechanisms of energy production fail and the bacteria fail to thrive.

At high concentrations, these effects can be so abrupt as to kill the organisms, but at clinically used doses, only bacteriostatic effects are generally observed. Overall, Gram-positive bacteria are generally more susceptible and, as with polymyxin B, the pore formation by gramicidin is influenced by the phospholipid composition of the bacterial membranes. MICs for common Gram-positive organisms are usually <30 μg/ml, with the effects being achieved in the presence of mucopurulent discharge.

The pharmacokinetics of topical ocular gramicidin do not appear to have been well studied. When used with other drugs, it can be expected to show good efficacy against Gram-positive organisms that are the common causes of blepharitis and blepharoconjunctivitis.

**Bacitracin zinc**

The drug, as its zinc salt, is taken up by bacteria and blocks any subsequent synthesis of certain structural components of the bacterial peptidoglycan cell walls. After exposure to bacitracin, the bacteria initially continue to thrive but slowly fail to assemble functional cell walls with a repeating N-acetyl-muraminic acid (NAM) unit.[20,21] The mechanism by which this effect is achieved is indirect in that bacitracin forms a Zn$^{2+}$ dependent complex with a special lipid carrier molecule (isoprenyl phosphate) present in the bacteria; the carrier is needed to transport the N-acetyl muraminic acid to cell wall assembly sites (Figure 8.4). Without this amino sugar incorporated in the cell walls, the bacteria are unable to resist any significant change in the osmolality (osmotic activity) of their surroundings and usually die as a result of osmotic cell rupture.

MICs for common Gram-positive organisms are usually between 0.001 and 5 U/ml,[18] with the effects being achieved in the presence of mucopurulent discharge. The ocular pharmacokinetics of bacitracin do not appear to have been studied in any detail. When used with other drugs, it can be expected to show good efficacy against Gram-positive organisms that are the

common causes of blepharitis and blepharo-conjunctivitis.[18]

**Trimethoprim**

Trimethoprim is an example of an inhibitor of intermediate metabolism in bacteria; it is an anti-infective drug.[21,22] The particular metabolic pathway that is important is that which converts p-aminobenzoic acid (PABA) to folic acid (dihydrofolate) and then to folinic acid (tetrahydrofolate); folinic acid is subsequently used in the synthesis of purine bases for DNA. An enzyme called dihydrofolate reductase is needed to reduce folic acid to tetrahydrofolate; trimethoprim is a potent inhibitor of this enzyme (Figure 8.5). A bacteriostatic action results from reduced nucleic acid synthesis needed for DNA. Its action will be reduced when mucopurulent discharge is present.

Trimethoprim is not used on its own because it can only exert weak bacteriostatic effects, but rather is used in combination with polymyxin B.[18] When used on its own, it would be expected to be more active against many common Gram-positive and Gram-negative bacteria, but shows very poor activity against *Pseudomonas* spp.

**Zinc sulphate**

Dilute solutions (i.e. *c* 0.25% w/v (Chapter 4)) of zinc sulphate are considered to have mild bacteriostatic action.[22] There was widespread use of this agent in the early years of this century in attempts to combat all sorts of eye infections. While such a claim was supported by the US Food and Drug Administration (FDA), equivalent clinical acceptance or evaluation in the UK appears restricted to anecdotal reports.

**Silver nitrate**

A 1% solution silver nitrate was once widely used to reduce the occurrence of acute conjunctivitis and blepharitis in very young infants, i.e. *ophthalmia neonatorum* or equivalent providing the causative organism was not chlamydia.[23] The solution would need to be prepared by a hospital pharmacy. Where it is still an elected procedure, treatments are more likely to be with chlortetracycline 0.5% ophthalmic,[24] or pharmacy-prepared erythromycin 0.5% ophthalmic ointment (see below).[25]

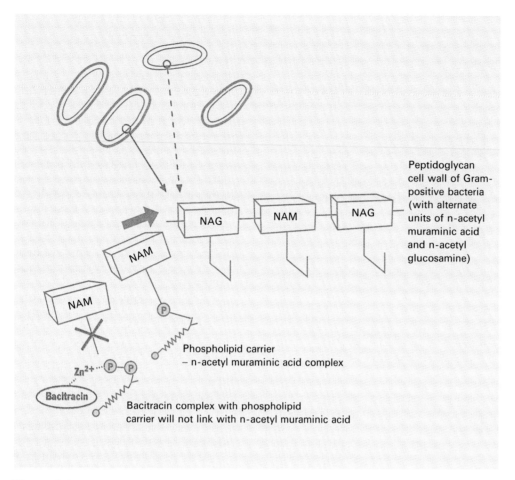

**Figure 8.4**
*Antibacterial action of bacitracin results from it entering cells and complexing with a phospholipid carrier molecule for cell wall subunit assembly.*

## Mechanisms of action of specific antibacterial drugs

A range of specific antibacterial drugs is available for ophthalmic use. These are all classified as broad-spectrum drugs in that they have a predictable action against a well-defined range of susceptible bacteria. These drugs are suitable for management of acute onset, moderate-to-severe bacterial infections of the external eye.

While a range of these drugs is available, some have become far more widely used than others simply because practitioners know they work in many cases. Such a confidence in outcome of therapy is based upon what is often called the 'shotgun' approach, where one or more pharmaceuticals is tried on a defined schedule of use; most external eye infections are resolved within a few days without there ever being any specific tests carried out for antibiotic sensitivity.

It should be stressed that such preferences for drug type or product should not be taken as true measures of efficacy since, regardless of how popular a product or drug is, efficacy can only be based on observing that a bacterial infection is rapidly attenuated.

Susceptibility is primarily determined by the drug effects on the bacteria in the laboratory (see above), but patient compliance with the recommended treatment regimen is still very important (see later). The selection of products will be determined in part by choices of antibacterial/corticosteroid products (see Chapter 9), and in part by experience of which products are found to be adequate to manage infections, especially unresponsive ones.

### Chloramphenicol

This broad-spectrum antibiotic is an inhibitor of protein synthesis in bacteria.[21,26] Protein synthesis involves sequential coupling (forming peptide bonds) of amino acid (AA)-tRNA precursor complex via a mRNA template (Figure 8.6). The synthesis occurs within the environment of two groups of globular microsomal protein aggregates called ribosomes.

Chloramphenicol blocks the effective incorporation of precursor molecules into synthesised protein (polypeptide) chains that would be assembled on larger (50S-sized) ribosomal protein aggregates of the bacteria as they prepare to divide.[21,26] Without adequate assembly of completed proteins, the bacteria fail to divide and the population fails to thrive. The drug binding to the ribosomes is of relatively low affinity and readily reversible so bacteriostatic effects are all that can be expected.

MICs for many common Gram-positive bacteria have been reported to be <16 μg/ml. The clinical pharmacokinetics have been well studied and it can be expected that, as a very lipophilic drug, it will have

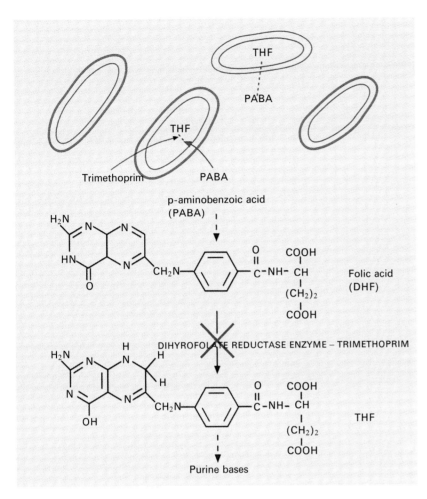

**Figure 8.5**
*Antibacterial action of trimethoprim results from its ability to inhibit a key enzyme (dibhydrofolate reductase) ultimately required for synthesis of DNA.*

excellent penetration through the corneal epithelium.[26,27] While peak concentrations of chloramphenicol of 2–6 μg/ml can be expected in the aqueous humour within an hour of presentation of eyedrops or ointment to the ocular surface, these values are generally below the MICs of many susceptible bacteria. Chloramphenicol ophthalmic is thus not indicated for severe infections.

Chloramphenicol, as ophthalmic eyedrops or eye ointment, has been successfully used for many years since its introduction in the 1950s.[26] It can be expected to show good efficacy against many bacteria that cause bacterial blepharoconjunctivitis, bacterial conjunctivitis and even mild-to-moderate cases of bacterial keratitis (especially where the keratitis is the secondary result of infections that originated at the eyelid margins or conjunctiva).[26,28]

Chloramphenicol is thus indicated for use to manage bacterial infections of the lids, conjunctiva and cornea, with the caveat that it cannot be expected to show good efficacy for established keratitis and corneal ulcers due to Gram-negative organisms such as *Pseudomonas*.

**Fusidic acid**
Fusidic acid, also known as fusidate sodium, is a protein synthesis inhibitor introduced in the 1960s. It has a narrow spectrum of action compared with chloramphenicol, but nonetheless has been repeatedly shown to have a similar efficacy to chloramphenicol when used to manage many common mild-to-moderate infections of the external eye.[29,30]

While it is generally not indicated for management of severe bacterial keratitis, it can be expected to have good efficacy

against a wide range of *Staphylococcus* strains that can be common causes of bacterial blepharoconjunctivitis.

Fusidic acid is structurally similar to the cephalosporin antibiotics, but has no specific effect on bacterial cell wall synthesis. The mechanism of action of fusidic acid is slightly different to chloramphenicol in that the drug binding to the 50S ribosome interferes with the continuing assembly of the polypeptide chain (see Figure 8.6); fusidic acid is also generally bacteriostatic.

Following topical application in the form of a slightly acid pH viscous gel (POM) Fucithalmic, Chapter 4, Figure 4.23), aqueous humour concentrations of around 0.5 μg/ml can be expected within a couple of hours and be sustained for many hours.[31] These levels are generally above the MICs reported for this drug against a range of susceptible Gram-positive and even some Gram-negative bacteria except *Pseudomonas* spp.[32]

**Aminoglycosides**
*Framycetin*
Framycetin is an aminoglycoside antibiotic that inhibits protein synthesis in bacteria, but by a slightly different mechanism to chloramphenicol or fusidic acid. In this case the drug binding is usually to the 30S subunit of the ribosome complex and prevents the actual initiation of protein synthesis (see Figure 8.6). The ribosome binding by aminoglycosides is usually high affinity and less reversible but this mode of action will still generally only lead to bacteriostatic effects.[33]

Resistance to framycetin and other aminoglycosides can arise as a result of mutations that alter the binding of the drugs to the ribosomal proteins. There is evidence that some bacteria are able to produce enzymes that degrade some aminoglycosides, the so-called aminoglycoside-modifying agents; the degraded antibiotic is no longer active so resistance develops.

The pharmacokinetics of ophthalmic framycetin do not appear to have been studied in detail, partly because it was superseded by the introduction of gentamicin, for which the pharmacokinetics have been well established (see below). Framycetin is indicated for use in the management of styes, blepharitis and bacterial conjunctivitis, corneal abrasions and even burns and peripheral ulcers, and can be expected

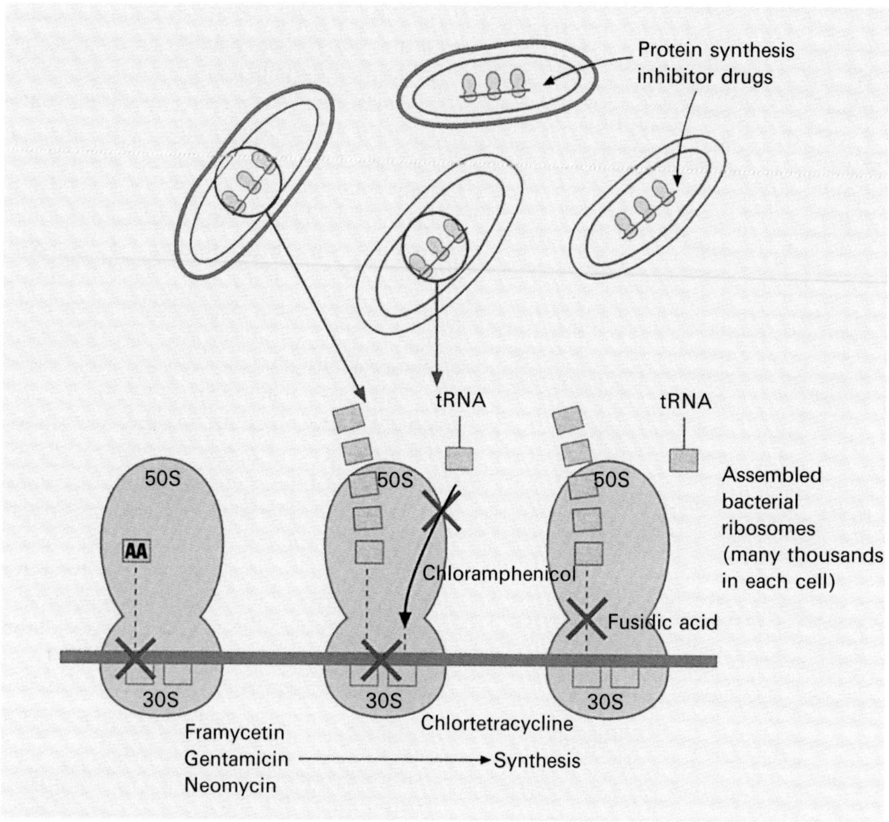

**Figure 8.6**
*Antibacterial action of protein synthesis inhibitors, such as chloramphenicol, results from their being able to interfere with the ribosome-sited assembly of new proteins required for bacterial growth.*

to have a similar spectrum of action to chloramphenicol.[34]

As an older aminoglycoside, the occurrence of resistant strains may be higher, although framycetin has been favourably compared with gramicidin for a wide range of bacteria isolated from the eye,[34] but less favourably against fusidic acid.[29]

*Gentamicin*

This is another aminoglycoside antibiotic which is thus also a protein synthesis inhibitor working at the same site as framycetin; it is also bacteriostatic in the first instance. However, the actual cellular uptake of aminoglycosides such as gentamicin into Gram-negative bacteria is partly dependent upon the ionic charge at the bacterial outer membrane surface. As such, the effective transfer of aminoglycosides into the bacterial cell can also result in a cancellation of this charge and thus secondarily affect the bacteria in addition to protein synthesis inhibition;[35] it is this cell membrane site that

ultimately results in gentamicin having a slow bactericidal action.

This specific uptake mechanism can be a major site of the development of resistance to aminoglycosides since the bacteria block the uptake of the drug into the cell. Pharmacokinetic studies using a 0.3% ophthalmic solution indicate that gentamicin will penetrate the cornea to a lesser extent than chloramphenicol,[36] but that peak concentrations of around 10 µg/ml will be achieved within one hour that are still around the MICs of 4–10 µg/ml for many susceptible bacteria.[37]

The lesser penetration can be overcome by using eyedrops or ointment more frequently for severe infections.

Gentamicin is indicated for use in many bacterial infections of the cornea and conjunctiva, including severe infections and ulcers susceptible to gentamicin.[38–40]

*Neomycin*

Neomycin is another broad-spectrum

aminoglycoside antibiotic very similar to framycetin and indicated for use in the management of styes, blepharitis and bacterial conjunctivitis, corneal abrasions and keratitis.[41,42]

**Tetracycline antibiotics, e.g. chlortetracycline**

This broad-spectrum antibacterial drug was also introduced in the 1950s and used in a wide range of bacterial infections of the external eye.[24] Its mechanism of action is also directed towards bacterial protein synthesis in which the drug binding to the 30 S ribosome interrupts protein synthesis, with a resultant bacteriostatic effect (see Figure 8.6).

At high concentrations, drugs such as chlortetracycline can be bactericidal but a special ointment formulation is needed to achieve such effects at the surface tissues; intraocular penetration of the topical tetracyclines is generally poor and inadequate for severe infections.

With the development of significant resistance and the introduction of more efficacious drugs, chlortetracycline ophthalmic ointment is now reserved for special uses only (see later).

**Fluoroquinolones**

Drugs such as ciprofloxacin, ofloxacin and lomefloxacin are newer antibacterial drugs that have similar broad-spectrum efficacy to gentamicin, but work by an entirely different mechanism. In this case, the drugs are taken up by the bacteria and bind to the active site of an enzyme (often collectively known as DNA gyrase) that is responsible for an organised disassembly and reassembly of the double chain helix of DNA that is required before DNA replication can occur.[43] As a result of inhibition of this enzyme activity, DNA synthesis is essentially blocked (Figure 8.7).

The relative penetration of fluoroquinolones such as ciprofloxacin and ofloxacin into the ocular tissues is poor compared with many other antibiotics,[44] and the aqueous humour concentrations of around 0.1 µg/ml are sometimes lower than MICs for organisms for which these drugs are primarily used,[7,45,46] e.g. *Pseudomonas* ulcers. However, where indicated for such use, the issue of complete tissue penetration through to the anterior chamber is less important, both because the barriers of the tissue are already severely compromised, and

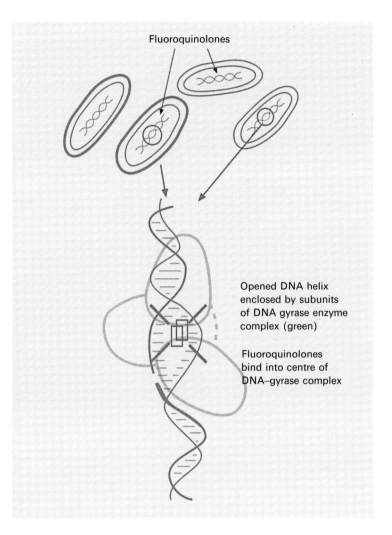

**Figure 8.7**
*Antibacterial action of fluoroquinolones results from their ability to inhibit a key enzyme (DNA gyrase) that is required for the replication of DNA to occur.*

discontinued in 1993. The major limitation to the use of the 'sulpha' drugs was that they would not be expected to show good efficacy if there was substantial muco-purulent discharge.

## Mechanisms of action of antiviral drugs for external eye disease

Infections of the external eye are not only caused by bacteria; viral and chlamydial infections may be encountered in certain areas at the same frequency as mild-to-moderate bacterial infections. Certain viral infections are amenable to either some local therapy or at least symptomatic treatment, while chlamydial infections unquestionably require oral antibiotic therapy. While selected viral infections and chlamydial infections of the eye may be considered the domain of secondary eye care, their management may be protracted (with recurrent infections developing) and so will be encountered in primary care.

Herpes simplex virus (HSV) and herpes zoster (HZ) infections can share similar symptoms and many ocular and periocular signs (especially in children).[50–52] However, zoster infections require oral antiviral drug therapy and need referral to an ophthalmologist and perhaps other specialists,[51] and may even require brief hospitalisation. HSV infections of the eyelid margins, the palpebral conjunctiva and cornea will often respond well to local antiviral drug therapy. Other viral eye infections, however, have no specific local therapy, e.g. epidemic keratoconjunctivitis (EKC) associated with adenovirus or enterovirus. These highly contagious infections require scrupulous management to prevent cross-infection,[22] but the actual management of the infection *per se* entails provision of symptomatic relief.

Ophthalmic antiviral drugs active against herpes simplex types 1 and 2 work by blocking the ability of the virus to replicate DNA. Acyclovir (also known as aciclovir) is actually a pro-drug in that the drug is largely ineffective against the virus, but will be biotransformed into the active form of the drug by an enzyme called thymidine kinase that is produced only in virus-infected corneal epithelial or conjunctival epithelial cells.[53,54] This biotransformation results in the production of a triphosphorylated derivative of the drug, acyclovir

adequate corneal tissue levels can be expected because the eyedrops are used very frequently.[46] Despite the rather different mechanism of action, resistance is already well known and can arise from mutations in the drug binding site on the gyrase enzyme for fluoroquinolones.[47]

Several other antibacterial drugs for ophthalmic use are probably well known but not generally available for use.

Another aminoglycoside antibiotic, tobramycin, was available for ophthalmic use until late 1997, when manufacture for UK distribution was discontinued. It was often used as the first alternative to gentamicin or as a first-choice drug by some practitioners, with an efficacy and spectrum of activity similar to gentamicin.[48]

The antibacterial drug erythromycin is a macrolide antibiotic introduced many years ago,[49] but is not generally marketed in the UK as an ophthalmic product. Erythromycin has a fairly broad spectrum of action through inhibition of bacterial protein synthesis, and may be prepared as an ophthalmic ointment by a hospital pharmacy for use in infections resistant to other antibiotics.

Finally, the original 'sulpha' (sulphonamide) drugs are still found in the printed version of the Optometrists' Formulary (as sulphacetamide sodium, mafenide and sulphafurazole) and although sulphacetamide 10% or 30% eyedrops could still probably be prepared by a hospital pharmacy, the last generally distributed product was

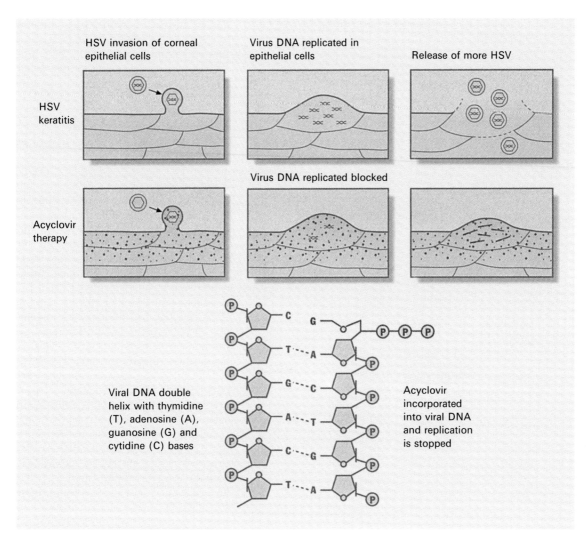

**Figure 8.8**
*Antiviral action of acyclovir only results after it is biotransformed by herpes virus-infected cells; the acyclovir derivative then inserts itself into the viral DNA and blocks further replication.*

triphosphate, that then acts as a nucleoside analogue specifically for the base deoxyguanosine.

The activated acyclovir exerts three effects. First it binds to an enzyme called viral DNA polymerase which then incorporates the acyclovir triphosphate into the DNA chain (Figure 8.8). Because of this incorporation, replication abruptly stops because no further bases can be added after acyclovir. As a result of binding to DNA polymerase, the enzyme is permanently inactivated.

The resultant DNA is fragmented and is non-functional as a template for subsequent mRNA and later protein synthesis, and so the virus fails to replicate.[54]

Acyclovir is not toxic to HSV *per se* but can be toxic to corneal epithelial cells.

## Mechanisms of action of other oral antibiotics for eye disease

Oral tetracyclines such as chlortetracycline or tetracycline may also be used for the long-term management of chronic and recurrent blepharitis, including that associated with recurrent meibomian gland infection,[24] or recurrent corneal erosions in conditions such as acne rosacea.[55] However, they are not recommended for routine use in children, and their use carries a general risk of

skin photosensitivity reactions (see Chapter 5).

Inclusion conjunctivitis, as caused by chlamydia infections for example, can be partly managed with several weeks' treatment with topical chlortetracycline (or erythromycin) ophthalmic ointment (or even eyewashes),[56] but several weeks' treatment with oral tetracyclines such as doxycycline,[57] or oral macrolides such as erythromycin[58] is generally recommended. Other oral macrolide antibiotics such as azithromycin can be effective for genital infections with a single massive dose, as opposed to chronic therapy with the other drugs,[59] but its efficacy for inclusion conjunctivitis is not well defined.

**Table 8.1  Factors to be considered in the management of mild-to-moderate infections of the external eye**

Opportunity to take a detailed history
Opportunity to evaluate the eye in detail
Recognition and appropriate initial diagnosis
of the cause of an infection:
- bacterial
- viral
- chlamydia
- fungal
- protozoan

Selection of a primary treatment regimen:
- selection of pharmaceutical product(s)
- selection of an appropriate daily treatment schedule
- selection of an appropriate duration of treatment

Provision of effective instructions to a patient
Provision of follow-up care

All these drugs block protein synthesis by chlamydia, so reducing the replication rate of this obligate intracellular virus-like organism (that is the cause of cellular 'inclusion' bodies, which are essentially encapsulated forms of the organism).

## Clinical strategies in anti-infective therapies for primary eye care

The effective management of mild-to-moderate infections of the external eye requires several factors to be considered (Table 8.1). These relate to the ability to take a detailed history, to undertake a provisional examination and diagnosis, the recognition of an infection (as opposed to other causes of a 'red eye'; see Chapter 6), selection of a primary treatment regimen (that requires both selection of a pharmaceutical product and an appropriate treatment schedule), provision of effective instructions to a patient and provision of follow-up care.

Bacterial infections of the eyelid margins often leave substantial encrustation on the eyelashes and bacterial infection of the conjunctiva is usually accompanied by white-yellow stringy/gummy mucopurulent discharge (although somewhat similar white and stringy mucous discharge can accompany some acute allergic reactions).

In bacterial infections, the extent of the mucopurulent discharge may be sufficient to make the lids stick together, especially overnight. In contrast, viral, chlamydial and fungal infections are more commonly accompanied by profuse tearing without discharge or encrustation, although foreign bodies and allergies must be ruled out as a cause too. The involvement of the conjunctiva may spread to the cornea.

Treatment with antibacterials is in order whenever an infection of the conjunctiva or corneal surface is suspected, or there has been a trauma or abrasion that might become infected, simply because of a compromised corneal or conjunctival epithelium (especially in ill or elderly patients). Hygiene measures may often be preferable in children, rather than antibacterial drug-based prophylaxis.

The outcome of treatment depends on whether the chosen therapy was actually effective against the pathogen, but starting therapies with a broad-spectrum antibiotic is the most widely used tactic, sometimes called the 'shotgun' approach. While it carries the inherent risk that the therapy will not be successful and will leave practitioners without samples of the microorganisms for culturing, the provision of adequate follow-up should all but ensure that mild-to-moderate infections do not get out of control (since the therapy can be switched to a different drug if not obviously responsive).

In severe infections, such samples for culture and antibiotic testing (to permit a 'bullet' therapy) need to be taken before treatment and then for the treatment to be started on an urgent basis. However, almost all mild-to-moderate conjunctival and eyelid infections can be successfully managed with broad-spectrum antibiotics without cultures.

As outlined above, all ophthalmic antibacterial products are not the same. In selecting a particular drug and pharmaceutical, probable efficacy should be considered. Equally important is the issue of allergies to ophthalmic antibiotics as these are the commonest reason for therapy being discontinued. Other issues include considering whether refrigeration for pharmaceuticals is available (e.g. for chloramphenicol eyedrops – see Chapter 4), considering how much discharge there is (since some ophthalmic antibacterial drugs may not be effective in infections where there is a lot of mucopurulent discharge, although ocular irrigation prior to application of the eyedrops can reduce this problem) and lastly to consider whether overnight antibacterial treatment ('coverage') will be necessary.

This coverage generally requires the use of ointments, but some antibacterial drug products are only available in solution form and do not have a companion ointment product for overnight coverage. It is perhaps easiest to prescribe from the same line of pharmaceuticals.

Any therapy for mild-to-moderate bacterial infections should be instigated at *q4h* or *q6h*. If the condition is more severe, all broad-spectrum ophthalmic antibacterial drugs can be administered *q3h* or even *q2h* during the first 24 hours. Ophthalmic gels can be used *bds*, i.e. *q6h* to *q8h* or 'morning and night'. The pharmaceuticals chosen and the prescribed regimen should always be noted in the patient's file. A reasonable regimen is 7–10 days with check-up (see below) and most infections should respond substantially over this period (providing the organism was sensitive to the drug or drugs used).

The check-up ensures that this response is occurring. An alternative strategy is to stipulate that the treatment should be until 2 or 3 days after the eye infection is no longer apparent and the eye is generally comfortable again. Wherever possible, an ointment should be used just before retiring, in addition to the *q4h* drops.

It should never be assumed that patients know how to use the drops or ointment containing an anti-infective; time should be taken to educate them on instillation/application, hygiene, storage and disposal of the pharmaceuticals. Reasonable effort should be made to ensure that the patient understands the importance of compliance. In uncertain cases it would be best to dispense an ointment.

Ideally, no patient should be prescribed anti-infective medications for eye infections without there being the opportunity for follow-up, i.e. it would be better to refer a patient to someone who can provide the follow-up rather than just dispensing tubes of POM Chloromycetin (or similar), and hoping the infection will be cured. Depending on the severity of the condition, the first follow-up should be at 24 or 48 hours. For moderate infections, a patient can usually be instructed at a second follow-up visit to continue therapy for one more week (or 2–3 days after the eye looks quiet again). In such cases where improvement is occurring, the follow-up could be via a telephone call with the intent of arranging a brief final check if considered appropriate. Obviously, if an eye appears worse on follow-up then appropriate changes in antibacterial therapy and referral, at the very least simply for cultures, is very important. In rare cases, it should be considered that the infection may not even be bacterial in nature, but due to a virus, chlamydia or a fungus.

## Pharmaceutical availability and use

The general-purpose antibacterial drugs are principally for mild-to-moderate infections of the conjunctiva and eyelids. These drugs (or drug combinations) are used for minor external eye and eyelid infections (including many childhood infections), and for prophylaxis against similar infections. Pharmacy medicines containing drugs such as propamidine (e.g. P Brolene and P Golden Eye, eyedrops and ointment) can be obtained by patients from a pharmacy, but any recommendations for the use of such products should be accompanied by a recommendation that (medical) attention be sought if the condition does not show signs of improvement within 2 days.

Where appropriate, the eyelid margins should be cleansed (but not excessively) and then the ointments worked into the lid margin (with a sterile cotton bud applicator) and the eyedrops used if the bulbar conjunctiva is affected as well. Nightly and morning use of the ointments should resolve the condition over 1–2 weeks for, although these drugs probably have little action on the bacteria inside the inflamed loci, they should stop the infection spreading; the lid cleansing (perhaps along with warm compress application for 5–10 minutes) should promote expression of the foci.

For general milder cases of bacterial blepharitis and blepharoconjunctivitis, there is no need to use a high-efficacy, potent broad-spectrum antibacterial drug. Adequate management can be achieved with often cheaper anti-infectives when used frequently at high doses, or when used as mixtures of several antibacterial drugs at low concentrations. Such products are not meant for use in any form of severe bacterial infection, especially when the condition is associated with substantial mucopurulent discharge or inflammation. Bacitracin and gramicidin provide coverage for Gram-positive organisms, while polymyxin B provides coverage against Gram-negative organisms.

Examples include combinations of polymyxin B with bacitracin (as POM Polyfax, 4 g tubes), trimethoprim and polymyxin B (as POM Polytrim, 5 ml bottles; as ointment in POM Polytrim Ointment, 4 g tubes), and combinations of polymyxin B, gramicidin and neomycin (as POM Neosporin, 5 ml bottles).

For cases of bacterial conjunctivitis, a range of broad-spectrum drugs is available. For example, chloramphenicol is widely available as 0.5% eyedrops (e.g. POM Chloromycetin Redidrops, 5 ml or 10 ml bottles; POM Sno Phenicol, 10 ml bottles). Numerous generic products containing chloramphenicol 0.5% for ophthalmic use are also available and inexpensive. Ointments containing 1% chloramphenicol are also available (e.g. POM Chloromycetin, 4 g tube) with a number of generic ointments marketed as well.

Fusidic acid is available as a unique viscous eyedrop at the 1% concentration, generally for *bds* usage. The viscous preparation is applied as if it were an ointment, but it then readily mixes with the tear film. The acid pH of the gel means that transient irritation (usually less than a minute) can be expected.[30] Partly due to the gel formulation, the drug can be effective even in the presence of large quantities of mucopurulent discharge from the eye.[32]

Several aminoglycosides are also available. Framycetin 0.5% eyedrops (Soframycin, 10 ml bottle) or as in ointment form (POM Soframycin, 5 g tube) are indicated for use in the management of styes, blepharitis and bacterial conjunctivitis, corneal abrasions and even burns and ulcers. Gentamicin is also widely available at the 0.3% concentration in eyedrops (e.g. POM Cidomycin Eyedrops, 8 ml bottle; POM Garamycin Eyedrops, 10 ml bottle; and POM Genticin Eyedrops, 10 ml bottle).

Neomycin is available but not commonly used. It is now only marketed in generic products (POM Neomycin, generic) of both the eyedrops (3500 units/ml) and ophthalmic ointment (3500 units/g). However, combination products with other antibiotics are available (see above).

Chlortetracycline is now only available in ointment form (e.g. POM Aureomycin, 3.5 g tubes) but its availability is questionable because of supply problems. It can be used for recurrent lid infections not responsive to other antibacterials.

While three fluoroquinolones are available (ciprofloxacin, ofloxacin and lomefloxacin) and can be expected to show equivalent efficacy to chloramphenicol for many cases of bacterial blepharoconjunctivitis and conjunctivitis,[60–62] it is illogical to use these potent drugs for such common conditions, unless there are good reasons for not using other drugs, e.g. lack of efficacy or development of allergies. The fluoroquinolones are primarily indicated for the management of severe keratitis and corneal ulcers, although lomefloxacin (POM Okacyn) is indicated for severe cases of acute bacterial conjunctivitis.[62]

Certain viral infections of the external eye can be managed easily and with a very favourable outcome, providing a prompt and correct diagnosis is made, that therapy is started and then adhered to. If diagnosed and treated early, first-time or recurrent (and uncomplicated) HSV infections of the conjunctiva and cornea require no more than a sustained course of antiviral drug therapy for effective resolution in 10–14 days.[51]

For HSV-related blepharitis and conjunctivitis and milder cases of keratitis, therapy should be initiated with acyclovir 3% ophthalmic ointment (POM Zovirax ophthalmic, 4.5 g tube). The dosing should be every 3 hours (*q3h*), especially for the first 24 hours at which time the regimen could be reduced to *q4h*. Such a treatment should be maintained for 7 days, preferably with examinations on days one, three and seven. If at 7 days significant improvement and re-epithelialisation is underway, the dosing can be maintained at *q4h* for a further 3–5 days and then discontinued. It is important that therapy be continued for a few days after resolution is clearly underway. If diagnosed early, treatment should not need to be continued for more than 14 days.[50,51,53]

Topical skin acyclovir ointments and creams are also available as pharmacy medicines and while these are definitely not for ophthalmic use, they may be indicated for topical skin use when the eye infections are associated with mouth ulcers or other skin lesions.

In contrast, EKC is not generally indicated for treatment with antiviral drugs. Management includes use of eyebaths and topical ocular decongestants (e.g. naphazoline 0.01% eyedrops) *prn* (to reduce lacrimation and promote ocular comfort). General hygiene measures to reduce the risk of cross-infection of other individuals is extremely important (including in the optometric practice!), although they are not always effective, especially at home. The total treatment period is not usually more than 2 weeks.

Since oral medications are required for inclusion conjunctivitis, and since it is so very important that the likely concurrent genital infections are also treated, patients with chlamydial conjunctivitis should be promptly referred to a sexually transmitted diseases (STD) clinic, not only for treatment but appropriate counselling.

## Adverse reactions to anti-infective therapies for external eye infections

The commonest 'ADR' consequential to the use of topical ocular antibacterial drug therapies is likely to be the development of an intolerance related to some form of allergic reaction to the drug or other ingredients of the pharmaceutical.[5] Allergies are more likely to be encountered with the aminoglycosides (e.g. neomycin) compared with other antibiotics, although even chloramphenicol can elicit a unique sensitisation,[63] especially if inappropriately used. Neomycin is considered by some to be the aminoglycoside that is most likely to precipitate allergic reactions of the lids and periocular skin. Patients reactive to neomycin may show cross-reactivity with other aminoglycosides such as framycetin and gentamicin. Gentamicin ophthalmic products may elicit local allergic or otherwise irritating reactions in patients sensitive to this, or neomycin and framycetin.

Whenever such a condition arises, the potentially offending drug or pharmaceutical should be promptly discontinued and, usually, another pharmaceutical started immediately. The consequences of an uncontrolled infection are likely to be far worse than some degree of discomfort associated with an inflamed eye. Side-effects such as general transient irritation are to be expected, partly because the eye is

already uncomfortable, and usually should not be a reason for discontinuing therapy. Should a punctate keratitis develop, however (e.g. with intensive use of gentamicin eyedrops), the therapy should be discontinued and other eyedrops used.

The use of any anti-infective drug always will carry the risk of overgrowth of non-responsive organisms, but the risk is minimised if appropriate follow-up examinations are carried out. Obviously, if an infection is not responding to therapy (and compliance is established) a patient should be referred to a corneal specialist, especially one in external eye diseases. This would be appropriate if the exogenous signs of an infection (e.g. mucopurulent discharge) continue to increase, or the endogenous signs (redness, oedema, or lesions) continue to develop despite hygiene and therapeutic intervention. The management of inflammation will be dealt with in Chapter 9.

Periodically, a particular drug or product will receive adverse press, especially from inappropriate use, e.g. chloramphenicol ophthalmic products. These are not intended for chronic use, nor even repeated regularly for short-term therapies. However, a small note in the directory listings for ophthalmic chloramphenicol states that an adverse drug reaction (ADR) is aplastic anaemia; this note also states that this reaction is rare.[64] Recent retrospective evaluations,[65] and commentary,[66] provide reassurance that the risk of aplastic anaemia from routine use of chloramphenicol ophthalmic products is extremely small.

Beyond a history of aplastic anaemia, it is not really possible to identify who might be at risk of developing such a potentially fatal adverse reaction which probably arises because of a pharmacogenetic difference in metabolism of this drug. Despite this, a few medical practitioners have expressed concern that the use of chloramphenicol eyedrops constitutes an unacceptable (and avoidable) risk, and that ophthalmic chloramphenicol should only be used when other ophthalmic antibiotics have failed to produce the desired effects.[22]

A guideline for the inappropriate use of chloramphenicol has been on some ophthalmic chloramphenicol products for more than 20 years,[22] and the latest assessments indicate that the risk of aplastic anaemia from chloramphenicol eyedrops

to be extremely small, i.e. <one in 200 000 patient prescription events.[65] This is consistent with most previous perspectives.[22]

## References

1 Baum J (1995) Infections of the eye. *Clin Infect Dis* **21**: 479–488.

2 McCloskey RV (1988) Topical antimicrobial agents and antibiotics for the eye. *Med Clin N Amer* **72**: 717–722.

3 Smith RE, Flowers CW (1995) Chronic blepharitis: A review. *CLAO J* **21**: 200–207.

4 Fisch BM (1991) Clinical management of eyelid disease. *Spectrum* February, pp. 40–50.

5 Stern GA, Klintworth DW (1989) Complications of topical antimicrobial agents. *Int Ophthalmol Clin* **29**: 137–142.

6 Kim HB, Okumoto M, Smolin G (1977) Quantitative antibiotic sensitivity determinations of *Staphylococcus aureus* isolated from eye cultures. *Arch Ophthalmol* **95**: 1065–1067.

7 Sutton SV, Franco RJ, Porter DA *et al.* (1991) D-value determinations are an inappropriate measure of disinfecting activity of common contact lens disinfecting solutions. *Appl Environ Microbiol* **57**: 2021–2026.

8 Richman J, Zolezio H, Tang-Liu D (1990) Comparison of ofloxacin, gentamicin, and tobramycin concentrations in tears and in vitro MICs for 90% of test organisms. *Antimicrob Agents Chemotherap* **34**: 1602–1604.

9 Elson WO (1945) The antibacterial and fungistatic properties of propamidine. *J Infect Dis* **76**: 193–197.

10 Hugo WB (1971) Amidines. In: *Inhibition and Destruction of the Microbial Cell* (Hugo WB, ed). Academic Press, New York, USA, pp. 121–136.

11 Valentine ECO, Edwards J (1944) Angular conjunctivitis treated with propramidine. *Lancet* **ii**: 753–754.

12 Wien R, Harrison J (1948) New antibacterial diamidines. *Lancet* **i**: 711–712.

13 Browning DJ, Foulkes GN (1984) Tear film pH in ocular disease. In: *The Preocular Tear Film* (Holly FJ, ed). Dry Eye Inst, Texas, USA, pp. 954–965.

14 Kagan BM, Krevsky D, Miller A *et al.* (1951) Polymyxin B and polymyxin E. Clinical and laboratory studies. *J Lab Clin Med* **37**: 402–414.

15 Storm DR, Rosenthal KS, Swanson PE (1977) Polymyxin and related peptide antibiotics. *Ann Rev Biochem* **46**: 723–763.

16 Bell TA, Slack M, Harvey SG *et al.* (1988) The effect of trimethoprim-polymyxin B sulphate ophthalmic ointment and chloramphenicol ophthalmic ointment on the bacterial flora of the eye when administered to the operated and unoperated eyes of patients undergoing cataract surgery. *Eye* **2**: 324–329.

17 Lund MH (1969) Colistin sulfate ophthalmic in the treatment of ocular infections. *Arch Ophthalmol* **81**: 4–10.

18 Bellows JG, Farmer CJ (1948) The use of bacitracin in ocular infections. *Am J Ophthalmol* **31**: 1211–1216.

19 Hunter FE, Schwartz LS (1967) Gramicidins. In: *Antibiotics* Vol. I (Gottlieb D, Shaw PD, eds). Springer-Verlag, New York, USA, pp. 642–648.

20 Weinberg ED (1967) Bacitracin, gramicidin and tyrocidine. In: *Antibiotics* Vol. I (Gottlieb D, Shaw PD, eds). Springer-Verlag, New York, pp. 244–247.

21 Gale E (1963) Mechanisms of antibiotic action. *Pharmacol Rev* **15**: 481–530.

22 Doughty MJ (1996) Diagnostic and therapeutic pharmaceutical agents for use in contact lens practice. In: *Clinical Contact Lens Practice* (Bennett ED, Weissman BA, eds). JB Lippincott, Philadelphia, USA Chapter 9, pp. 1–38.

23 O'Hara MA (1993) Ophthalmia neonatorum. *Pediat Clin N Amer* **40**: 715–725.

24 Salamon SM (1985) Tetracyclines in ophthalmology. *Surv Ophthalmol* **29**: 265–275.

25 Bell TA, Sanderstrom KI, Gravett MG *et al.* (1987) Comparison of ophthalmic silver nitrate and erythromycin ointment for prevention of natally-aquired chlamydia trachomatis. *Sex Transm Dis* **14**: 195–200.

26 Leopold IH, Nichols AC, Vogel AW (1950) Penetration of chloramphenicol U.S.P. (Chloromycetin) into the eye. *Arch Ophthalmol* **44**: 22–36.

27 Beasley H, Boltralik JJ, Baldwin HA (1975) Chloramphenicol in aqueous humor after topical application. *Arch Ophthalmol* **93**: 184–185.

28 Roberts W (1951) Topical use of chloramphenicol in external ocular infections. *Am J Ophthalmol* **34**: 1081–1088.

29 Dirdal M (1987) Fucithalmic in acute conjunctivitis. Open, randomized companion of fusidic acid, chloramphenicol and framycetin eye drops. *Acta Ophthalmol* **65**: 129–133.

30 Horven I (1993) Acute conjunctivitis. A comparison of fusidic acid viscous eye drops and chloramphenicol. *Acta Ophthalmol* **71**: 165–168.

31 Hansen S (1985) Intraocular penetration of fusidic acid with topical Fucithalmic. *Eur J Drug Metabl Pharmacokin* **10**: 329–331.

32 Taylor PB, Burd EM, Tabbara KF (1987) Corneal and intraocular penetration of topical and subconjunctival fusidic acid. *Br J Ophthalmol* **71**: 598–601.

33 Prober C (1984) Antimicrobial agents which affect synthesis of cellular proteins. In: *Principles of Medical Pharmacology* (Kalant H, Roschlau WHE and Seller EM, eds). 4th edn. Department of Pharmacology, Faculty of Medicine, University of Toronto, Canada.

34 Mahajan VM, Angra SK (1977) In vitro activity of framycetin and gentamicin against microbes producing ocular infection. *Indian J Ophthalmol* **24**: 13–17.

35 Bryan LE, Kwan S (1983) Roles of ribosomal binding, membrane potential and electron transport in bacterial uptake of streptomycin and gentamicin. *Antimicrob Agents Chemotherap* **23**: 835–845.

36 Furgiuele FP (1967) Ocular penetration and tolerance of gentamicin. *Am J Ophthalmol* **64**: 421–426.

37 Magnuson R, Suie T (1970) Clinical and bacteriologic evaluation of gentamicin ophthalmic preparations. *Am J Ophthalmol* **70**: 734–738.

38 Bras JF, Coyle-Gilchrist MM (1968) Gentamicin in conjunctivitis and keratitis. *Br J Ophthalmol* **52**: 560–561.

39 Halasa AH (1967) Gentamicin in the treatment of bacterial conjunctivitis. *Am J Ophthalmol* **63**: 1699–1702.

40 Gordon DM (1970) Gentamicin sulfate in external eye infections. *Am J Ophthalmol* **69**: 300–306.

41 Lopez SP (1954) Topical use of neomycin in ophthalmology. *Antibiot Chemotherap* **4**: 1189–1195.

42 Saraux H (1956) La collyre a la neomycine dans les conjonctivites. *Sem Hosp Paris* **32**: 1504–1506.

43 Shen LL, Kohlbrenner WE, Weigle D *et al.* (1989) Mechanism of quinolone inhibition of DNA gyrase. *Biochemistry* **28**: 2973–2978.

44 Donnenfeld ED, Scrier A, Perry HD *et al.* (1994) Penetration of topically applied ciprofloxacin, norfloxacin, and ofloxacin into the aqueous humor. *Ophthalmology* **101**: 902–905.

45 Thomson KS, Sanders CC, Hayden ME (1991) In vitro studies with five quinolones: evidence for changes in relative potency as quinolone resistance rises. *Antimicrob Agents Chemotherap* **35**: 2329–2334.

46 Diamond JP, White L, Leeming JP *et al.* (1995) Topical 0.3% ciprofloxacin, norpfloxacin, and ofloxacin in treatment of bacterial keratitis: a new method for comparative evaluation of ocular drug penetration. *Br J Ophthalmol* **79**: 606–609.

47 Wolfson JS, Hooper DC (1989) Flouroquinolone antimicrobial agents. *Clin Microbiol Rev* **2**: 378–424.

48 Laibson P, Michaud R, Smolin G *et al.* (1981) A clinical comparison of tobramycin and gentamicin sulphate in the treatment of ocular infections. *Am J Ophthalmol* **92**: 836–841.

49 Querengesser EI, Ormsby HL (1955) Ocular penetration of erythromycin. *Can Med Assoc J* **72**: 200–202.

50 Wishart MS, Darougar S, Viswalingam ND (1987) Recurrent herpes simplex virus ocular infection: epidemiological and clinical features. *Br J Ophthalmol* **71**: 669–672.

51 Liesegang TJ (1988) Ocular herpes simplex infection: Pathogenesis and current therapy. *Mayo Clin Proc* **63**: 1092–1105.

52 Liesegang TJ (1991) Diagnosis and therapy of herpes zoster ophthalmicus. *Ophthalmology* **98**: 1216–1229.

53 Jackson WB, Breslin CW, Lorenzetti DWC *et al.* (1984) Treatment of herpes simplex keratitis: comparison of acyclovir and vidarabine. *Can J Ophthalmol* **19**: 107–111.

54 Wagstaff AJ, Faulds D, Goa KL (1994) Aciclovir. A reappraisal of its antiviral efficacy, pharmacokinetic properties and therapeutic efficacy. *Drugs* **47**: 153–205.

55 Hope-Ross MW, Chell PB, Kervick GN *et al.* (1994) Oral tetracycline in the treatment of recurrent corneal erosions. *Eye* **8**: 384–388.

56 Darougar S, Viswalingam E, El-Sheikh H *et al.* (1981) A double-blind comparison of topical therapy of chlamydial

ocular infection. *Br J Ophthalmol* **65**: 549–552.

57 Carta F, Zenetti S, Pinna A *et al.* (1994) The treatment and follow up of adult chlamydial opthalmia. *Br J Ophthalmol* **78**: 206–208.

58 Patamasucon P, Rettig PJ, Faust KL *et al.* (1982) Oral versus topical erythromycin for chlamydial conjunctivitis. *Am J Dis Child* **136**: 817–821.

59 Lode H, Borner K, Koeppe P *et al.* (1996) Azithromycin – review of key chemical, pharmacokinetic and microbiological features. *J Antimicrob Chemotherap* **37** (suppl C): 1–8.

60 Bron AJ, Rizk SNM, Baig H *et al.* (1991) Ofloxacin compared with chloramphenicol in management of external ocular infection. *Br J Ophthalmol* **75**: 675–679.

61 Bloom PA, Leeming JP, Power W *et al.* (1994) Topical ciprofloxacin in the treatment of blepharitis and blepharoconjunctivitis. *Eur J Ophthalmol* **4**: 6–12.

62 Aguis-Fernandez A, Patterson A, Fsadni M *et al.* (1998) Topical lomefloxacin versus topical chloramphenicol in the treatment of acute bacterial conjunctivitis. *Clin Drug Invest* **15**: 263–269.

63 Verin MM, Sekkat A, Morax S (1972) Chloramphenicol en instillation ophthalmique et riske de sensibilisation generale. *Bull Soc Ophthalmol Fr* **72**: 365–370.

64 Ammus S, Yunis AA (1989) Drug-induced red cell dyscrasias. *Blood Reviews* **3**: 71–82.

65 Lancaster T, Swart A, Jick H (1998) Risk of serious haematological toxicity with use of chloramphenicol eye drops in a British general practice database. *Br Med J* **316**: 667.

66 Doughty MJ (1998) Reassurance on ocular chloramphenicol. *Optician* **215**: 15.

# 9
# Ophthalmic corticosteroids: management of the ocular inflammatory response

Overview of the ocular inflammatory response
Mechanisms of action of corticosteroids
Indications for use of topical ophthalmic corticosteroids
Ophthalmic corticosteroid products, selection and use
Combination corticosteroid-antibacterial products
Therapeutic uses of cycloplegics for ocular inflammation
Contraindications for ophthalmic corticosteroid use
Precautions for ophthalmic corticosteroid use
Potential ocular ADRs from systemic corticosteroid use

## Introduction

The inflammatory response of the tissues of the eye is the result of a series of complex actions effected by a range of inflammatory mediators.[1,2] Almost any stress, insult or damage to the external eye can be expected to result in conjunctival vasodilation and release of mediators such as histamine, prostaglandins and other substances;[1,2] a range of eye washes, astringents, topical and oral antihistamines and mast cell stabilisers can be used to manage this level of the inflammatory response (see Chapter 6).[3,4]

Another group of aspirin-like medication called non-steroidal anti-inflammatory drugs (NSAIDs) can also be used as eyedrops in some other countries in Europe, Canada and the USA to manage mild-to-moderate inflammatory responses associated with allergic reactions, but these drugs are not currently indicated for such uses in the UK.

In more substantial cases of inflammation of the external eye, stronger anti-inflammatory drugs are needed and this is the indicated use for ophthalmic corticosteroids. With the appropriate diagnosis and availability of follow-up to monitor the efficacy of the therapy, short-term usage (i.e. 1–3 weeks) of ophthalmic corticosteroid products represents a most effective way of not only combating the inflammation and preventing further tissue trauma, but providing substantial patient comfort.

In many cases, the adjunct use of either topical antibacterial products (to reduce the risk of secondary infection) and cycloplegic drugs (to promote comfort and reduce other sequelae of the inflammatory response) is also indicated.

## Mechanisms of action of corticosteroids

From the perspective of ocular inflammation, corticosteroid drugs can simply be considered as anti-inflammatory agents, although these drugs can exert a wide range of other effects in the body, especially when administered by routes other than the conjunctiva. One group of mineralocorticosteroids serves to regulate kidney function, while glucocorticosteroids control tissue glucose homeostasis and energy balance.

When presented to the eye in the form of eyedrops, suspensions or ointments, the action of the glucocorticosteroids is local and while some systemic absorption of these corticosteroids is inevitable after such conjunctival presentation (see Chapter 2), evidence of clinically significant systemic effects following such absorption is minimal.[5,6] When corticosteroids are used, especially systemically, there is always a chance that the natural immune system can be suppressed as a result of their action on the inflammatory processes.

Corticosteroids (especially hydrocortisone, also known as cortisol) are normally present in the circulation of the body and bind to specific receptors in cells throughout the body. Cortisol is released whenever there is stress, injury or infection,[2,7] and

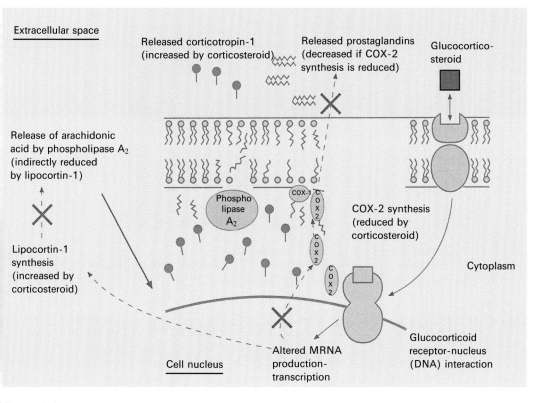

**Figure 9.1**

*Schematic diagram to illustrate the corticosteroid-induced anti-inflammatory mechanism involving increased synthesis of lipocortin-1 (to suppress phospholipase A2 activity) and decreased synthesis of COX-2 (cyclo-oxygenase-2 activity). The net result is reduced production of pro-inflammatory mediators such as the prostaglandins.*

this general statement is presumably applicable to the eye, even though there are few specific studies on this.[8,9]

However, with respect to the eye, it can be noted that plasma levels of hydrocortisone can be expected to show a diurnal variation, and the vascular systems of the eye (including the secretion of the aqueous humour, and thus intraocular pressure) is probably regulated by these cyclical changes.[10]

It is important to note that ophthalmic corticosteroids were once widely referred to as only 'palliative' (cover-up) drugs since it was considered that they did little actually to counter the inflammatory response. It is now widely recognised that glucocorticosteroids are true therapeutic drugs that block the development of the inflammatory response.[11] This recognition is really an extension of an acceptance that natural glucocorticosteroids serve to dampen the normal inflammatory response of the body so that it does not proceed out of control.

With this perspective, it is reasonable to consider that the extent of development of ocular tissue oedema will thus depend upon natural glucocorticosteroid levels, and the addition of corticosteroids as medications is thus a supplement to a natural mechanism and regulatory cycle. However, recognising that glucocorticosteroids can 'cover-up' the signs of tissue disease is still important since practitioners should be aware that any ongoing differential diagnosis needs to take into account the palliative effects.

In short, this should translate to an important clinical guideline in that ophthalmic glucocorticosteroid use, even if brief, should be carefully supervised, i.e. with regular follow-up examinations to check both for efficacy and for any unwanted reactions. When used in this way, ophthalmic glucocorticosteroids are extraordinarily effective and safe therapeutic drugs.

The receptors and mechanisms of action of corticosteroids are unusual (Figure 9.1). The receptors are located inside the cells so that the corticosteroids have to enter the cells to achieve an effect. All cells, including

the 'inflammatory cells' (e.g. macrophages, leucocytes etc), appear to contain glucocorticosteroid receptors and most evidence suggests that these receptors, once bound with corticosteroids, become intimately associated with the nucleus of mammalian cells. Once bound to their receptor, glucocorticosteroids are able to interact with DNA in such a way as to alter the rates of synthesis of certain gene products.

There are probably many such products relevant to the inflammatory process but the ones best understood at this time are for a peptide hormone called lipocortin-1 (also now known as annexin-1),[11] and certain enzymes responsible for synthesis of pro-inflammatory mediators such as the prostaglandins, i.e. the enzyme prostaglandin synthetase-2 (known as cyclo-oxygenase-2, or COX-2).[12] COX-2 is down-regulated by glucocorticosteroids so lesser quantities of prostaglandins are produced to mediate tissue inflammation. The lipocortin-1 has actions on enzymes and inflammatory cells. It can act as an anti-inflammatory agent by reducing the activity of two key enzymes called phospholipase A2 and nitric oxide synthase.[13,14]

The mechanism(s) is poorly defined but is probably mediated at the gene transcription level rather than the lipocortin-1 actually acting as an inhibitor of the enzymes (as once widely thought). The cell membrane-sited activity of phospholipase A2 is an essential initial step in the synthesis of another group of chemicals that causes the tissue inflammatory response, including a fatty acid called arachidonic acid. With reduced phospholipase A2 activity, a continued tissue stress does not result in the release of arachidonic acid and, as a result, lower levels of prostaglandins are produced (since arachidonic acid is converted into prostaglandins by the action of cyclo-oxygenase enzymes) (see Figure 9.1).

Lipocortin-1 is also actually released from glucocorticoid-activated cells and is thought also to play a role to reduce recruitment of inflammatory cells to the site of tissue stress etc.[15]

Cellular activity of nitric oxide (NO) synthase is essential for the production of the potent vasodilator nitric oxide and so reduced NO-synthase activity means lesser vasodilation and thus reduced movement of inflammatory cells from the circulation into the tissues (of the eye for example).[2,16]

Glucocorticosteroids also reduce the tissue expression of unique cell surface proteins such as intracellular adhesion molecule-1 (ICAM-1) that assist in the movement of inflammatory cells across the surface of the eye,[2] but the mechanism underlying this effect is uncertain.

Most glucocorticosteroids used as therapeutic drugs are synthetic corticosteroids but mimic the action of hydrocortisone. The use of these synthetic corticosteroids should thus reduce the extent of the inflammatory response and their use is essential to control true tissue inflammation, as opposed to acute or chronic vasodilation which can be managed with other drugs (see Chapter 6).

For primary eye care, a useful guideline is that the use of local (ocular) corticosteroid therapy should be short term (e.g. up to 3 weeks) and designed to provide much-needed relief of inflammation that is unlikely to resolve solely through the protracted use of direct- or indirect-acting antihistamines and/or vasoconstrictors (Chapter 6). Such a use of ocular corticosteroids should be distinguished from uses

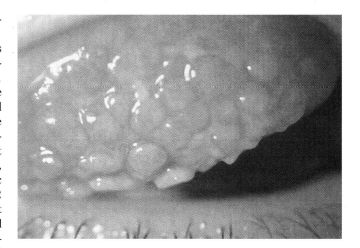

**Figure 9.2**
*Cobblestone-like papillae in advanced vernal keratoconjunctivitis (Reproduced with permission from* Clinical Ophthalmology. A Systematic Approach *(1999) by J. J. Kanski).*

for moderate-to-severe inflammatory conditions, and following ocular surgery. None of these more substantial conditions would be likely to respond to direct- or indirect-acting antihistamines and/or vasoconstrictors in the first instance anyway.

This distinction can essentially be made as being inflammatory conditions of the external vs the internal eye. The rationale behind the judicious clinical use of topical synthetic corticosteroids is both directly to attenuate the local tissue reactions (including vasodilation, oedema, pain etc), and prevent extended disruption of the vascular system (that could lead to significant tissue infiltration and damage that can be caused by macrophages and other white blood cells). To achieve the latter goal, it is essential that there is early corticosteroid intervention.

## Indications for use of topical ophthalmic corticosteroids

Ophthalmic corticosteroid preparations are indicated for use whenever there is inflammation present, or a risk of this developing. The use of the ophthalmic corticosteroids should directly reduce leakiness of the vasculature of the anterior uvea, and reduce the rate of migration of white blood cells into the ocular tissues. Topical ophthalmic corticosteroids are available as eyedrops or ointments, often in combination with anti-infective drugs.

Corticosteroids take a relatively long time to act (days, rather than hours or minutes) because their receptors are intracellular and the mechanisms of action are indirect. Equally importantly, rather a long time period is also required for the effects of corticosteroid therapy to cease after the administration of these drugs has been stopped. Therefore, for clinically useful effects to occur, corticosteroids might need to be given for a few days before any effect is really apparent, and this represents a difficult therapeutic strategy.

From a primary eye care perspective, there are a number of relatively common conditions for which careful use of topical ocular corticosteroid therapy would be indicated and appropriate.

Perhaps highest on the list are conditions that arise from chronic irritation of the palpebral or bulbar conjunctiva associated with repeated exposure to allergens, or even chemical vapours wherein substantial papillae develop on the tarsal plate, e.g. vernal keratoconjunctivitis (Figure 9.2). A combination of aggressive therapy with mast-cell stabilisers and periods of judicious local steroid use would prevent the condition from developing to this extent.[9,17] Similarly, early steroid intervention should reduce the chance of later corneal complications such as a shield ulcer developing.

Another common condition, hopefully on the decline, is the development of severe papillary conjunctivitis as a result of what is now recognised as a consequence of over-wear of dirty and/or poorly fitted contact lenses (Figure 9.3). The aetiology

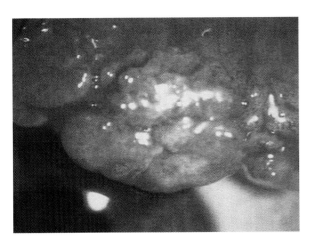

**Figure 9.3**
*Severe conjunctivitis associated with giant papillae (grade IV) on tarsal plate (Reproduced with permission from* Clinical Ophthalmology. A Systematic Approach *(1999) by J. J. Kanski).*

may be predominantly chemical (as a reaction to deposits on the lens) or mechanical but the consequence is probably the same.[18,19] Early intervention such as planned replacement of lenses may reduce the rate of onset of this condition but, once developed, it may well need more than a temporary discontinuation of lens wear to resolve.

As therapeutic options and with early intervention, mast-cell stabiliser use *qds* for 2–4 weeks may be adequate to resolve the papillae and mean that corticosteroid use is not required, i.e. the use of drugs such as sodium cromoglycate should be considered as an important steroid-sparing therapy. However, when presenting at a substantial (severe) level, a short course (e.g. 1–2 weeks) of corticosteroid eyedrops will hasten the recovery process to a level where non-corticosteroid strategies can be effective (see Chapter 6).[18] These strategies may also be maintained during corticosteroid therapy if used initially.

In other cases, it may be more the eyelid margins that are affected, whether this is associated with chronic blepharitis (which needs to be managed as well) or developing concurrent with systemic inflammatory diseases, e.g. ocular rosacea (Figure 9.4). In this advanced example, inflammatory tissue has developed across the bulbar conjunctiva including scar tissue. Early intervention with corticosteroids (along with appropriate systemic management of the rosacea) should reduce the chance of such a condition developing.[20–23]

Similarly, chronic infection of the eyelids

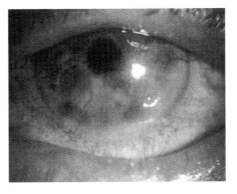

**Figure 9.4**
*Eyelid margin oedema, meibomian gland dysfunction, corneal neovascularisation, limbal pannus formation and mild epitheliopathy in advanced rosacea keratitis (Reproduced with permission from* Clinical Ophthalmology. A Systematic Approach *(1999) by J. J. Kanski).*

with *Staphylococcus* can lead to the development of marginal corneal infiltrates or even peripheral 'catarrhal' ulcers (Figure 9.5) as a result of an allergic and toxic reaction to products released by the bacteria (often referred to as 'exotoxins') or the white blood cells (e.g. eosinophil cationic proteins).[2] In this case, at least at earlier stages, judicious use of corticosteroid ointments should reduce the development of both the corneal infiltrates and the substantial eyelid margin oedema.

Chronic meibomian gland dysfunction as an entity in itself or associated with conditions such as chronic blepharitis or

rosacea, can also result in very unwanted chronic oedema of the eyelid margins and some superficial corneal epithelial involvement should be expected as well. Therefore, indications for careful topical ocular corticosteroid use logically extend to superficial punctate keratitis (SPK) of almost any aetiology providing there is no evidence of a true ulcer developing which could ultimately extend to an active stromal inflammatory condition.[20,21]

It is a matter of debate which of the various inflammatory conditions of the sclera and anterior chamber should be considered suitable for primary eye care, although the case can arguably be made that many of these sorts of conditions are likely to be diagnosed as superficial inflammations and or infections by general medical practitioners. It should also be noted that the inclusion of inflammatory conditions of the sclera as primary eye care and within the realm of optometric practice is by no means new.

A non-steroidal anti-inflammatory drug called oxyphenbutazone (Tanderil eye ointment) could be used for episcleritis,[22] and initial 'emergency' treatment by an optometrist would have been possible until the commercial product was withdrawn from the market.

These types of conditions should generally be acute or subacute in their history and a number of hallmark signs and symptoms should be looked for. A relatively painful eye that shows sectorial (regional/localised) superficial injection and local chemosis well away from limbus is likely to be caused by chronic irritation, including eye rubbing in response to symptoms, and diagnosed as simple episcleritis of unknown aetiology (Figure 9.6).

Examination should rule out the presence of any form of foreign body and then a short course (e.g. 1–2 weeks) of corticosteroid eyedrops should effectively reduce this superficial local inflammation. Local corticosteroid use may well be the first line of therapy, although non-steroidal strategies (e.g. cold compresses, topical ocular vasoconstrictors/antihistamines, and/or mast-cell stabilisers) can provide some symptomatic relief for this sort of condition (see Chapter 6).

If the injection is extending more around the entire bulbar conjunctiva and closer to the limbus, then a deeper-lying and more generalised inflammation such as scleritis or anterior uveitis should be suspected.

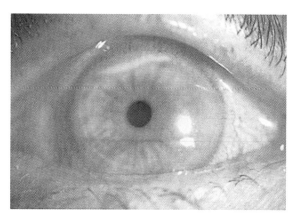

**Figure 9.5**
*Marked confluent peripheral infiltrates and generalised superficial punctate keratitis (SPK) in marginal keratitis associated with eyelid margin-related staphylococcal exotoxin release (catarrhal ulcer) (Reproduced with permission from* Clinical Ophthalmology. A Systematic Approach *(1999) by J. J. Kanski).*

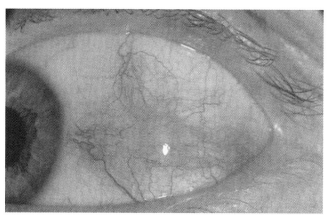

**Figure 9.6**
*Localised superficial conjunctival vasodilation and oedema of temporal bulbar conjunctiva associated with simple sectorial episcleritis (Reproduced with permission from* Clinical Ophthalmology. A Systematic Approach *(1999) by J. J. Kanski).*

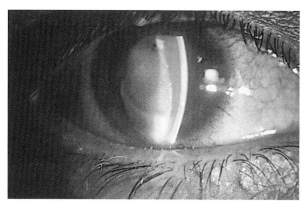

**Figure 9.7**
*Moderated generalised conjunctival vasodilation and perilimbal/ciliary vasodilation (injection) in acute anterior uveitis with accompanying corneal oedema (Reproduced with permission from* Clinical Ophthalmology. A Systematic Approach *(1999) by J. J. Kanski).*

Such an affected eye (Figure 9.7) will probably be painful and accompanying signs to the circumciliary injection include corneal oedema and an obvious reaction in the anterior chamber.

A cut-off for severity of the presenting condition can well be made on the basis of a narrow-beam slit-lamp assessment of the anterior chamber for flare (protein and cells) (Figure 9.8). The protein leaks from substantially dilated deeper-lying blood vessels (of the anterior uvea) and the cells are actually white blood cells that have migrated out of the vasculature and into the aqueous humour. In the example (Figure 9.8), the grade IV flare is not the result of a trivial inflammation.

Such an anterior uveitis is unlikely to respond adequately to a short course of even potent local corticosteroid therapy and is unlikely to be considered as primary eye care, especially because it is often associated with an exacerbation of a systemic inflammatory disease such as rheumatoid arthritis.

Adequate medical treatment of the systemic condition (including use of systemic non-steroidal anti-inflammatory drugs and systemic corticosteroids) is thus an essential part of the management of such severe conditions.

When an inflammation of the external surface of the eye or especially the anterior uvea develops, the pupil is likely to be slightly or substantially miotic and some anterior chamber reaction should be evident. These signs can be helpful in distinguishing such inflammatory causes of ciliary injection from those with a totally different aetiology and which definitely should not be treated with corticosteroids. An example is illustrated in Figure 9.9 of marked generalised injection over a substantial portion of the bulbar conjunctiva associated with a slightly dilated pupil and modest corneal oedema arising as a result of angle-closure; such an eye would likely be relatively painful (but not necessarily so) and the pupil sluggish in light response. The key differential will however be identification of the (markedly) elevated IOP.[24]

## Ophthalmic corticosteroid products, selection and use

Ophthalmic corticosteroids and the different products can be ranked approximately in order of increasing anti-inflammatory

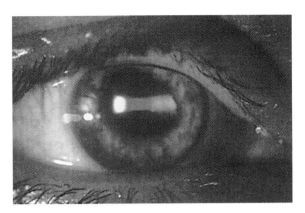

**Figure 9.8**
*Aqueous chamber protein (flare) and cell (4+ grade) in moderate-to-severe anterior uveitis; note distal scleral involvement as well (Reproduced with permission from* Clinical Ophthalmology. A Systematic Approach *(1999) by J. J. Kanski).*

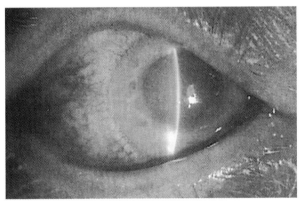

**Figure 9.9**
*Ciliary injection, corneal oedema and dilated pupil associated with acute congestive primary angle-closure glaucoma (Reproduced with permission from* Clinical Ophthalmology. A Systematic Approach *(1999) by J. J. Kanski).*

action. This is important because, as with the systemic use of corticosteroids, ophthalmic corticosteroid selection is largely done on the expected drug potency rather than its concentration or dosing regimen.

For mild-to-moderate inflammations, mild-to-moderate potency corticosteroids are indicated for periodic use; for severe inflammations, moderate-to-strong corticosteroids are indicated for periodic or intensive use. There is no one scale of potency that is agreed upon by all, especially because different derivatives of the corticosteroids may have a different bioavailability (see Chapter 2) as a result of different rates of tissue and cell penetration, and can be used at different dosing regimens.[10,22,23,25–28] A relative scale of one to five is adopted here as a guideline to why the different products can be expected to show different efficacy and this is the general basis for selection of a particular product. All ophthalmic corticosteroid preparations in the UK are prescription-only medicines (POM), and most are preserved with benzalkonium chloride.

## Eyedrops and ointments containing hydrocortisone

This steroid, as its acetate derivative, has a relative ophthalmic anti-inflammatory activity of one. It can be used for relatively superficial non-infectious inflammatory conditions of the lids or conjunctiva where there is no major defect or signs of ulceration. These hydrocortisone products are marketed at the 1% strength in eyedrops (POM Hydrocortisone, generic, 10 ml bottle) or at the 1% and 2.5% strength in ointment form (POM Hydrocortisone, generic, 3 g tubes). It is the ointments that have the most useful application for eyelid conditions.

## Eyedrops containing clobetasone

This steroid, as its butyrate derivative, has a relative ophthalmic anti-inflammatory activity of two. It is generally indicated for milder inflammatory conditions, although can be used more aggressively as a postoperative steroid. It is available at the 0.1% concentration in eyedrops (e.g. POM Cloburate, 10 ml bottles). It is useful for management of inflammatory conditions predominantly affecting the superficial conjunctiva (e.g. chronic seasonal allergic conjunctivitis) rather than the eyelids or where the inflammation is more localised.

## Eyedrops or ointments containing betamethasone

This steroid, as its sodium phosphate salt, has an ophthalmic anti-inflammatory activity of three to four. It is thus indicated for use in moderate inflammatory conditions of the lids, conjunctiva, corneal epithelium and localised more superficial inflammations of the sclera (although it can be used more aggressively as a postoperative steroid). It is available as eyedrops as a 0.1% suspension (e.g. POM Betnesol, 10 ml bottle, and POM Vista-Methasone, 5 ml and 10 ml bottles) and also in an ophthalmic ointment at the 0.1% concentration (POM Betnesol, 3 g tube).

## Eyedrops containing fluorometholone

This steroid, as its base, has an ophthalmic anti-inflammatory activity of five, but is used in the UK at a low concentration (0.1%), so is generally indicated for mild-to-moderate inflammations of the conjunctiva and corneal epithelium when a rapid response is deemed appropriate. Fluorometholone is available as eyedrops at 0.1% concentration (POM FML Liquifilm, 5 ml or 10 ml bottles).

Other marketed ophthalmic corticosteroids include dexamethasone and prednisolone but these are more widely used postsurgically to manage inflammation developing as a result of surgery. Dexamethasone, as its sodium phosphate or sodium metasulphobenzoate derivatives, has a relative ophthalmic anti-inflammatory activity of three, but is used intensively for severe inflammations. It is available as eyedrops at the 0.1% concentration in 5 ml or 10 ml bottles as (e.g. POM Maxidex), and in unit-dose form (POM Minims Dexamethasone).

A combination product with the antibiotic framycetin is however useful for eyelid conditions (see later).

Prednisolone is probably the most widely used ophthalmic corticosteroid for moderate-to-severe and deeper-sited inflammations, including postoperative use. It is available at two strengths and as different derivatives, with the sodium phosphate derivatives considered to have a relative ophthalmic anti-inflammatory activity of three or four, while the acetate derivative is thought by some to have slightly superior anti-inflammatory activity.[29]

Prednisolone is available as eyedrops at the 0.5% concentration (e.g. POM Predsol, 10 ml bottle; POM Minims Prednisolone, unit-dose) as well as eyedrops at the 1% concentration (e.g. POM Pred Forte, 5 ml and 10 ml bottles). The 1% product is a suspension rather than a solution of the drug, and needs to be shaken before use.

A new type of ophthalmic steroid is rimexolone, now available as POM Vexol. It is considered to have anti-inflammatory efficacy, when used as a 1% ophthalmic suspension, equivalent to prednisolone acetate 1%, but generally, needs to be used on a more intensive schedule or for longer periods of time.[30]

In other countries, other ophthalmic corticosteroids are available, such as medrysone and lotoprednol.

An ophthalmic steroid is selected based on its potency, i.e. how much anti-inflammatory activity is needed, allowing for slight differences in strength of the preparations. For inflammations of the external eye, dosing for topical ocular corticosteroid should be started at *q4h* or *q6h*, whether this be the application of a 0.5–1 cm ribbon of ointment along the eyelid margins or instillation of eyedrops into the lower cul-de-sac. With the types of conditions outlined above, ophthalmic corticosteroid preparations should not need to be used for extended periods, and an opinion has been published that this period of treatment should not be longer than 3 weeks.[31]

After starting corticosteroid therapy and on reassessment at 48 to 72 hours, if definite signs of improvement are not evident then the condition should be considered unresponsive and referred to a specialist. The temptation of continuing corticosteroid treatment when early promising signs are not evident should be avoided, especially because the aetiology may be far more serious.

With signs of improvement, a decision will need to be made whether the period of *qds* treatment should be continued *bds* for 1 or 2 weeks. After these two respective time periods, the use of the corticosteroids should be reduced. This is referred to as 'tapering' the therapy, e.g. to *bds* and then *od* over 2–3 days. Treatment with ophthalmic corticosteroids should not be abruptly stopped unless a severe adverse reaction develops.

For acute conditions, depending on the severity of the condition, the follow-up assessments should best be made 2 and 7 days and then every 4–7 days thereafter until substantial resolution of the condition has occurred (as shown by diminution of symptoms and unambiguous reduction of the signs of inflammation). The ocular assessment should cover general inspection (including eyelid eversion and inspection), biomicroscopy (including evaluation of the anterior chamber for any reaction/flare/cells, etc) and evaluation of the pupil/iris (especially for signs of acute inflammatory reaction).

Patient records should include notes as to the magnitude of the oedema and should be made such that some degree of objectivity is possible in deciding the degree of resolution or otherwise of any corneal oedema and other reactions at both central and more peripheral sites. Notes on patient compliance and satisfaction with the therapy can also be useful.

## Combination corticosteroid–antibacterial products

The main use for ophthalmic corticosteroids in primary eye care should be for non-infected inflammatory conditions. However, a range of combination products containing corticosteroids and a broad-spectrum antibiotic (see Chapter 8) are available. For commonly encountered conditions, there are compelling reasons why combination therapy with such anti-bacterial drugs and corticosteroids should be considered.[32] These are for short-term management of inflammatory disease associated with bacterial infections of the eyelids or conjunctiva, providing there is evidence that the bacterial infection is under control (and not in a developing phase). Short periods of adjunct use of corticosteroids should thus be considered appropriate for chronic, mild-to-moderate, inflammation of the eyelids where there is a risk of bacterial infection, or a bacterial infection is actually present, i.e. cases of severe allergic conjunctivitis, blepharoconjunctivitis, vernal conjunctivitis, acne rosacea and select cases of episcleritis.

However, starting treatment with combination products should be avoided when there is a moderate-to-severe inflammatory condition of the anterior segment where the aetiology of the infection is uncertain (see contraindications, below). A case can be made that intensive corticosteroid–antibacterial drug therapy is essential in inflammatory diseases where there is a risk of bacterial infection (e.g. herpes zoster infections, post-trauma keratitis from burns, chemical injuries, significant postoperative keratitis or after the removal of deep or penetrating foreign bodies, or following many types of ocular surgery), but this is not primary eye care.

An ointment combination product for hydrocortisone was available until mid-1996, but its current availability for human use is questionable (e.g. POM Chloromycetin–Hydrocortisone, 4 g tubes). The combination can obviously also be achieved by concurrent use of hydrocortisone eyedrops or ophthalmic ointment with chloramphenicol 0.5% eyedrops (e.g. POM Sno-Phenicol, 10 ml bottle) or 1% ointment (e.g. POM Chloromycetin, 4 g tubes). With the lower potency of hydrocortisone, such a combination would best be limited to milder eyelid and conjunctival conditions, although consideration should always be given to a special risk of patient sensitisation to chloramphenicol with repeated use (see Chapter 8).[4,33]

Such a combination therapy should be started at *qds* and continued until the inflammation resolves. It should then be tapered to once daily or at bedtime, and the therapy with the chloramphenicol continued for 2 or 3 more days.

Corticosteroid combination products for dexamethasone are available that contain framycetin 0.5% and gramicidin 0.005% with dexamethasone 0.05% (POM Sofradex; eyedrops 10 ml and ointment 5 g). The combination could also be achieved with framycetin 0.5% eyedrops (10 ml bottle) or ointment (5 g tube) (both POM Soframycin), and dexamethasone 0.1% eyedrops (POM Maxidex).

The ointment combinations would likely have most use in primary eye care for conditions where a little more anti-inflammatory efficacy was considered necessary. In such cases, the ointment could perhaps only be used at bedtime, to supplement a daytime *qds* therapy with the antibacterial for cases of blepharoconjunctivitis instead of the combination product being used during the day. Combination therapy should be continued until the inflammation resolves and use of the combination product is tapered, and then simply stopped, and the antibacterial product used for a further 2 or 3 more days.

Clobetasone, betamethasone and fluorometholone are available in combination eyedrops with the broad-spectrum antibiotic neomycin, e.g. POM Cloburate-N (neomycin 0.5% with clobetasone 0.1%, 10 ml bottles), POM Betnesol-N (neomycin 0.5% with betamethasone 0.1%, 10 ml bottles), POM Vista-Methasone (neomycin 0.5% with betamethasone 0.1%, 5 ml and 10 ml bottles), POM FML-Neo (neomycin 0.5% with fluorometholone 0.1%, 5 ml bottles).

## Therapeutic uses of cycloplegics for ocular inflammation

When even superficial inflammations of the external eye occur, some internal inflammation can develop as well, with the ultimate result being an increase in the protein levels in the anterior chamber and some cells being present. Even a slight anterior chamber reaction can be associated with considerable discomfort (pain) and this calls for special use of mydriatic-cycloplegic drugs. These will help relieve the discomfort and may be used prophylactically in eyes considered at risk of developing inflammation or once the inflammation has developed.

The mydriatic-cycloplegic does not necessarily need to be concurrent with corticosteroid use and it may well be argued that the mydriatic-cycloplegic is a suitable alternative to corticosteroids in conditions such as ocular surface abrasion or following removal of superficial foreign bodies.

For episcleritis or simple scleritis, the condition can be painful and adjunct therapy with a mydriatic-cycloplegic drug is essential to reduce this pain (perhaps with supplementary systemic analgesics).

The pain relief is achieved as a result of a relaxation of the ciliary body and also because the mydriatic-cycloplegic should also reduce vasodilation of the inflamed tissues and reduce the development of oedema, etc. The cycloplegic effects reduce the 'tugging' sensation that accompanies inflammation and spasms of muscle contraction. In addition to promoting comfort, their use is for preventive care even in acute or subacute conditions affecting the external coat of the eye, since the ensuing inflammation could result in adhesions developing between the miotic pupil and the lens capsule. These posterior synechiae, if uncorrected, can lead to unwanted iris atrophy or damage.

The mydriatic-cycloplegic should usually be started at either the first signs of intraocular inflammation, or after the external trauma to the eye, and should be continued for as long as the intraocular inflammation or risk of inflammation is present. In selecting to use a mydriatic-cycloplegic, the same type of precautions that apply to their use as diagnostics should be considered.[34] These include the risk of anterior chamber angle-closure (bearing in mind that eyes that develop posterior synechiae are at even greater risk of a secondary angle-closure due to pupil block) and of IOP (see later). The extent of the mydriasis and cycloplegia is important for such therapies and the dosing regimen should be consistent with the degree of ocular pigmentation, i.e. the darker the eye, the greater the dosing needed.

Since the mydriatic action serves to counter both the inflammation-related miosis (due to release of certain prostaglandins and substance P) and the inflammation-related contraction and oedema of the ciliary body, the regimen of use of the mydriatic-cycloplegic may only produce slight mydriasis (as opposed to the pupil being miotic) but can also produce substantial mydriasis.

Patient age as well as ocular pigmentation will likely play an important role in determining the extent of the cycloplegia, with the overall goal being more simply to relax the muscles inside the eye, rather than try to achieve maximal effects. The duration of the use of the mydriatic-cycloplegic will depend on the condition being managed, but for primary eye care, a few days is usually all that would be required, e.g. after a significant abrasion.

The usual drug is atropine 1% available as POM Atropine (generic) or POM Isopto Atropine eyedrops (10 ml or 5 ml bottles respectively); a POM Minims Atropine Sulphate (unit-dose eyedrops) could also be used for short-term management. It should be used at bedtime for mild-to-moderate cases and twice-daily for moderate cases. The cycloplegic should be the last of the drops instilled into the eye since these eyedrops tend to sting more than others; reflex tearing will wash the corticosteroid and/or antibacterial drugs out from the eye, thus reducing the efficacy. A five-minute interval, between antibiotic/corticosteroid eyedrops and the mydriatic-cycloplegic, is reasonable.

The use of homatropine is an alternative, but the available multiple-use pharmaceuticals only contain 1% or 2% homatropine, rather than 5% (e.g. POM Homatropine eyedrops; generic, 10 ml bottles). These drug doses and regimens are necessary since the pharmacokinetics of these products may be substantially different in the inflamed eye compared with the non-inflamed eye.

## Contraindications for ophthalmic corticosteroid use

Significant complications can develop if ophthalmic corticosteroids are inappropriately used, either in terms of the eye conditions or with respect to follow-up.[27] The potential for these complications can often be forwarded as reasons why ophthalmic corticosteroids should not be used in primary eye care, yet need not occur if certain precautions are taken (Table 9.1).

Starting therapy with corticosteroids is contraindicated when there is a concurrent active herpes simplex virus (HSV) infection since the corticosteroid use can exacerbate an active HSV keratitis and lead to the development of severe stromal disease (Figure 9.10). Part of the initial eye examination should thus include use of fluorescein and biomicroscopy along with an appropriate history to rule out HSV as a cause of the problems; the use of fluorescein and biomicroscopy should also be included at check-up visits to search for the presence of even the smallest corneal surface lesion (surface or dendritic).

Some also recommend that other viral infections should also not be managed initially with corticosteroids. Similarly, initial corticosteroid use is contraindicated for red eyes developing as a result of fungal, protozoan or active tuberculosis infections;

**Table 9.1 Contraindications (C/I) and specific precautions (S/P) for initiating ocular therapy topical corticosteroid products**

*C/I* (see note 1)
- Known allergy to drug or any ingredient of the pharmaceutical
- Narrow-angle glaucoma
- Uncontrolled ocular hypertension
- Active viral infections of the cornea and conjunctiva (see note 2)
- Active fungal infections of the cornea and conjunctiva
- Active protozoan infections of the cornea and conjunctiva (see note 3)
- Active tubercule infections of the cornea and conjunctiva
- Purulent infections (especially of unknown aetiology)

*S/P*
- Monitor for secondary infection developing
- Avoid prolonged use in pregnancy
- Limit use in infants

Note 1 – the safety and efficacy of concurrent topical corticosteroid eyedrop (or ointment) use while continuing with contact lens wear has not been established for any UK-marketed products. As a result, concurrent corticosteroid use for CL wearers has to be listed as contraindicated, by order of the Committee on the Safety of Medicines. How it might be applied to the therapeutic use of soft (bandage) contact lenses has yet to be defined, although it is not a recommended use.[4]

Note 2 – e.g. as evidenced by any form of patterned epithelial break (dendritic ulcer) typically associated with herpes simplex virus (HSV) infection; other forms of viral infection such as adenovirus or enterovirus may show no more than punctate epitheliopathy and clear guidelines in relation to corticosteroid use are not available.

Note 3 – the CSM does not apparently acknowledge the existence of protozoan infections of the cornea, or perhaps does not distinguish between fungal and protozoan infections.

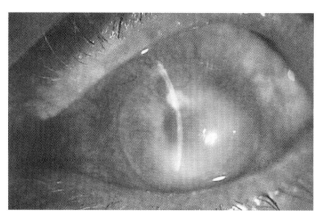

**Figure 9.10**
*Gross stromal necrotic keratitis resulting from uncontrolled stromal invasion of herpes simplex virus (HSV) (Reproduced with permission from* Clinical Ophthalmology. A Systematic Approach *(1999) by J. J. Kanski).*

history of the development of the red eye will be the primary diagnosis here (and the condition referred to a specialist if there is any uncertainty).

As with HSV infections, the initial concurrent steroid may exacerbate an active fungal or protozoan infection of the eye (*Acanthamoeba* protozoan infection in contact lens wearers is a current well-known concern), but any history of a known vegetative injury to the eye, hot-tub use, or home-made saline solutions for contact lens wear should be taken as sufficient circumstantial evidence to refer such an eye rather than start treatment for the inflammation in primary care.

The increased risk factors relate to fungal contamination.

Similarly, any patient with ocular inflammation and a history of tuberculosis (Tb) infections requires a comprehensive work-up, which should include evaluation of the status of their past Tb-related problems (and re-instigation of, or changing of medications for Tb).

At the primary care level, topical corticosteroid would be contraindicated in any form of corneal disease with significant stromal involvement, e.g. significant generalised or localised central or peripheral thinning ('corneal melting' associated with major inflammatory disease), and any form of stromal partial thickness ulcerating lesions. Corticosteroid use could exacerbate these types of conditions.

## Precautions for ophthalmic corticosteroid use

Corticosteroid therapy of the eye should be contraindicated in purulent bacterial infections simply because it is far more important to get the infection under control quickly rather than worrying about inflammation; mydriatic–cycloplegic use can provide some comfort. Furthermore, the corticosteroid therapy, while an essential part of management of tissue inflammation, can also interfere with the body's natural defence to such infections as well as mask the appearance of the bacterial infections, so any indication that the infection is getting worse may not be so evident.

The presence of purulent discharge makes assessment of the eye in terms of the anti-inflammatory efficacy and the potential development of any adverse reactions more difficult; this difficulty can be limited by restricting use.

Corticosteroid therapies will do nothing to combat a bacterial infection in terms of slowing bacterial replication or preventing their spread, and the opposite can in fact be argued in that concurrent corticosteroid therapy may exacerbate an infection (partly because the corticosteroids may reduce ocular surface re-healing). Similarly, longer-term steroid use could increase the risk of overgrowth of pathogens that are non-responsive to antibiotic drugs, including both resistant strains of bacteria, opportunistic bacteria, fungi, etc. The risk is present partly because the corticosteroid therapy masks the development of a secondary infection.

On lowering steroid dose, and particularly upon discontinuation of the corticosteroid therapy, signs and symptoms may get a little worse for a day or so, especially if there is still a mild degree of infection present. Should this occur, it should be an antibacterial therapy that is intensified, not the corticosteroid.

## Potential ocular ADRs from corticosteroid use

Three major potential complications of ophthalmic corticosteroid therapy are often presented as reasons why they should either only be used for short periods or not used at all. These complications relate to poor wound healing of the corneal or conjunctival epithelium, the risk of elevated IOP and the risk of development of cataracts.[6,27] However, providing follow-up is made available and achieved, these risks are minimal.

Follow-up assessment with suitable biomicroscopy, as opposed to a cursory unaided external eye examination, should readily identify the presence of a non-healing lesion on the ocular surface; steroid therapy should be tapered immediately and prophylactic measures such as use of lubricating artificial tears and/or more viscous antibacterial eyedrops started to provide comfort and promote healing.

IOP elevation is a most unlikely consequence of short-term use of ophthalmic corticosteroids for the types of conditions being considered in this chapter. However, the possibility cannot be ignored and a measure of IOP should be considered as essential before the start of ophthalmic corticosteroid therapy to identify any patient who might already have elevated intraocular pressure and thus be at risk for greater elevations.[35] As a precautionary measure, IOP should be reassessed at the time corticosteroid therapy is discontinued 2–3 weeks later.

Listings for ophthalmic corticosteroids in *MIMS* and the *BNF* include a caution about the possibility of an adverse drug reaction (ADR); this may be referred to as 'steroid glaucoma' or raised intraocular pressure. Corticosteroid eyedrops can increase IOP to unacceptable levels and this needs to be checked for at each patient assessment.

The reason for this is that a small percentage of the population (exact number uncertain) displays an unusual ocular response to topical ocular corticosteroids

in that, over a period of 2–3 weeks, their IOP increases to more than 25 mmHg and can increase much further if corticosteroid therapy is not reduced.[36] The response has been attributed to the presence of a unique set of special glucocorticosteroid receptors in the trabecular meshwork. The older corticosteroids (e.g. hydrocortisone) and those indicated for and used aggressively to manage moderate-to-severe inflammations (e.g. dexamethasone or prednisolone) may increase IOPs more than other corticosteroids (e.g. clobetasone or fluorometholone).

This potential difference in ADR-response magnitude does not mean that patients prescribed clobetasone or fluorometholone eyedrops do not need to be monitored regularly. The patients that develop an increased IOP are thought to have a genetic predisposition to such corticosteroid-induced ocular hypertension; these patients are known as 'steroid responders'. The IOP should return to normal levels over 1–2 weeks when corticosteroid therapy is tapered and discontinued. Therefore, IOP must be monitored periodically, especially in longer-term therapy, to identify these responders; 'periodically' can be translated to every 10–14 days.

It needs to be recognised and emphasised that systemic administration of corticosteroids can also produce ocular hypertension and some high-risk groups have been identified,[37,38] just as they have for local therapy.[39] Furthermore, with corticosteroid preparations for the nose, skin and mucous membranes (haemorrhoids) now widely available as pharmacy medicines, one surely has to accept that such uses pose a higher risk than short-term use of ophthalmic corticosteroids.

The development of cataracts, specifically posterior subcapsular cataracts (PSSC), following short-term use of topical ophthalmic corticosteroids, is an extraordinarily unlikely outcome, although cases have been reported following long-term indiscriminate, and what would now be considered inappropriate, use.[6,31,40] As with the risk of IOP elevation, oral corticosteroid use poses a much greater risk of PSSC development,[41] and especially in some high-risk patient groups,[42–45] e.g. those with renal failure. A number of cases of PSSC development associated with systemic prednisolone therapy have been reported to the College of Optometrists.[46] Patients on long-term systemic corticosteroid therapy

should probably have checks for cataracts every 6 months. As with ocular hypertension, there has also been recent attention to the significant cataractogenic potential of nasal or topical skin corticosteroid use,[41,47–49] and again the relative risk from the indiscriminate use of pharmacy medicines must be considered as greater than short-term supervised use of ophthalmic corticosteroids.

## References

1 Millichamp NJ, Dziezyk J (1991) Mediators of ocular inflammation. *Prog Vet Comp Ophthalmol* **1**: 41–48.

2 Doughty MJ (1998) The pathological response of the anterior eye. *Optometry Today* Feb 13, pp. 28–32.

3 Doughty MJ (1997) A guide to ophthalmic pharmacy medicines in the United Kingdom. *Ophthal Physiol Opt* **17** (suppl 1): S2–S8.

4 Doughty MJ (1996) Diagnostic and therapeutic pharmaceutical agents for use in contact lens practice. In: *Clinical Contact Lens Practice* (Bennett ED, Weissman BA, eds). JB Lippincott, Philadelphia, USA Chapter 9, pp. 1–38.

5 Nursall JF (1965) Systemic effects of the topical use of ophthalmic corticosteroid preparations. *Am J Ophthalmol* **59**: 29–30.

6 Wilson FM (1979) Adverse external ocular effects of topical ophthalmic medications. *Surv Ophthalmol* **24**: 57–88.

7 Munck A, Guyre PM, Holbrook NJ (1984) Physiological functions of glucocorticosteroids in stress and their relation to pharmacological actions. *Endocrine Rev* **5**: 25–44.

8 Streilein JW, Wilbanks JW, Cousins SW (1992) Immunoregulatory mechanisms of the eye. *J Neuroimmunol* **39**: 185–200.

9 Abelson MB, Scaefer K (1993) Conjunctivitis of allergic origin: immunologic mechanisms and current approaches to therapy. *Surv Ophthalmol* **38**: 115–132.

10 McCarty GR, Schwartz B (1991) Increased plasma noncortisol glucocorticoid activity in open-angle glaucoma. *Invest Ophthalmol Vis Sci* **32**: 1600–1608.

11 Buckingham JC, Flower RJ (1997) Lipocortin 1: a second messenger of

glucocorticoid action in the hypothalamo-pituitary-adrenocortical axis. *Molec Med Today* July, pp. 296–301.

12 Newman SP, Flower RJ, Croxtall JD (1994) Dexamethasone suppression of IL-1-beta-induced cyclooxygenase-2 expression is not mediated by lipocortin-1 in A549 cells. *Biochem Biophys Res Comm* **200**: 931–939.

13 Goppelt-Strebe M (1997) Molecular mechanisms involved in the regulation of prostaglandin biosynthesis by glucocorticosteroids. *Biochem Pharmacol* **53**: 1389–1395.

14 Wu C-C, Croxtall JD, Perretti M et al. (1995) Lipocortin 1 mediates the inhibition by dexamethasone of the induction by endotoxin of nitric oxide synthase in the rat. *Proc Natl Acad Sci USA* **92**: 3473–3477.

15 Getting SJ, Flower RJ, Perretti M (1997) Inhibition of neutrophil and monocyte recruitment by endogenous and exogenous lipocortin 1. *Br J Pharmacol* **120**: 1075–1082.

16 Meijer F, Tak C, Van Aheringen NJ et al. (1996) Interaction between nitric oxide and prostaglandin synthesis in the acute phase of allergic conjunctivitis. *Prostaglandins* **52**: 431–446.

17 Lee Y, Riazman MB (1997) Vernal conjunctivitis. *Immunol Allergy Clin N Amer* **17**: 33–51.

18 Trocme SD, Raizman MB, Baitley GB (1992) Medical therapy for ocular allergy. *Mayo Clin Proc* **67**: 557–565.

19 Mondino BJ, Salamon SM, Zaidman GW (1982) Allergic and toxic reactions on soft contact lens wearers. *Surv Ophthalmol* **26**: 337–344.

20 Aragones JV (1973) The treatment of blepharitis: a controlled double blind study of combination therapy. *Ann Ophthalmol (Chic)* **5**: 49–52.

21 Driver PJ, Lemp MA (1996) Meibomian gland dysfunction. *Surv Ophthalmol* **40**: 343–367.

22 Watson PG, McKay DA, Clemett RS et al. (1973) Treatment of episcleritis. A double-blind trial comparing betamethasone 0.1 per cent, oxyphenbutazone 10 per cent, and placebo eye ointments. *Br J Ophthalmol* **57**: 866–870.

23 Duke-Elder S, Duthie OM, Foster J et al. (1951) A series of cases treated locally by cortisone. *Br J Ophthalmol* **35**: 672–694.

24 Greenidge KC (1990) Angle-closure glaucoma. *Int Ophthalmol Clin* **30**: 177–186.

25 Baba S, Mishima H, Okimoto M et al. (1983) Plasma steroid levels and clinical effects after topical application of betamethasone. *Graefe's Arch Clin Exp Ophthalmol* **220**: 209–214.

26 Kadom AH, Forrester JV, Williamson TH (1986) Comparison of the anti-inflammatory activity and effect on intraocular pressure of flouromethalone, clobetasone butyrate and betamethasone phosphate eyedrops. *Ophthal Physiol Opt* **6**: 313–315.

27 Rubin B, Palestine AG (1989) Complications of corticosteroid and immunosuppressive drugs. *Int Ophthalmol Clin* **29**: 159–172.

28 Pilz A, Roy D, Hesse M et al. (1991) Die Wirkung von Fluorometholon auf den intraokularen Druck – eine multizentrische Studie. *Folia Ophthalmol* **16**: S 12–15.

29 Sousa FJ (1991) The bioavailability and therapeutic effectiveness of prednisolone acetate vs. prednisolone sodium phosphate: a 20-year review. *CLAO J* **17**: 282–284.

30 Foster CS, Alter G, De Barge LR et al. (1996) Efficacy and safety of rimexolone 1% opthalmic suspension vs. 1% prednisolone acetate in the treatment of uveitis. *Am J Ophthalmol* **122**: 171–182.

31 Butcher JM, Austin M, McGaillard J, Bourke RD (1994) Bilateral cataracts and glaucoma induced by long term use of steroid eyedrops. *Br Med J* **308**: 43–44.

32 Thomas RK, Melton NR (1994) A review of common ophthalmic antibacterial and corticosteroid-antibacterial combination drugs. *Optom Clin* **2**: 45–57.

33 Doughty MJ (1998) Reassurance on ocular chloramphenicol. *Optician* **215**: 15.

34 Doughty MJ (1997) Pupillary dilation. The standard for delivery of primary eye care. *Optometry Today* Dec 12, pp. 24–28.

35 Godel V, Feiler-Ofry V, Stein R (1972) Systemic steroids and ocular fluid dynamics. II. Systemic versus topical steroids. *Acta Ophthalmol* **50**: 664–676.

36 Akingbehin T (1986) Corticosteroid-induced hypertension. *J Toxicol Cut Ocular Toxicol* **5**: 45–53.

37 Tripathi RC, Kirschner BS, Kipp M et al. (1992) Corticosteroid treatment for inflammatory bowel disease in pediatric patients increases intraocular pressure. *Gastroenterology* **102**: 1957–1961.

38 Opatowsky I, Feldman RM, Gross R et al. (1995) Intraocular pressure elevation associated with inhalation and nasal corticosteroids. *Ophthalmology* **102**: 177–179.

39 Jain IS, Gill MM (1969) Effect of topical steroids on intraocular pressure in young diabetics. *J All-India Ophthalmol Soc* **17**: 95–98.

40 Yablonski ME, Burde RM, Kolker AE et al. (1978) Cataracts induced by topical dexamethasone in diabetics. *Arch Ophthalmol* **96**: 474–476.

41 Urban RC, Cotlier E (1986) Corticosteroid-induced cataracts. *Surv Ophthalmol* **31**: 102–110.

42 Ticho U, Durst A, Licht A et al. (1997) Steroid-induced glaucoma and cataract in renal transplant recipients. *Israel J Med Sci* **13**: 871–874.

43 Limaye SR, Pillai S, Tina LU (1988) Relationship of steroid dose to degree of posterior subcapsular cataracts in nephrotic syndrome. *Ann Ophthalmol(Chic)* **20**: 225–227.

44 Fournier C, Milot JA, Clermont M-J, O'Regan S (1990) The concept of corticosteroid cataractogenic factor revisited. *Can J Ophthalmol* **25**: 345–347.

45 La Manna A, Polito C, Todisco N et al. (1994) Corticosteroid therapy, cataracts and chronic glomerulopathy – a survey on 23 patients. *Ann Ophthalmol (Chic)* **26**: 131–133.

46 Edgar DF, Gilmartin B (1997) Ocular adverse reactions to systemic medication. *Ophthal Physiol Opt* **17** (suppl 2): S1–S7.

47 Costagliola C (1989) Cataracts associated with long-term topical steroids (letter). *Br J Dermatol* **120**: 472–473.

48 Fraunfelder FT, Meyer SM (1990) Posterior subcapsular cataracts associated with nasal or inhalation corticosteroids. *Am J Ophthalmol* **109**: 489–490.

49 Cumming RG, Mitchell P, Leeder SR (1997) Use of inhaled corticosteroids and the risk of cataracts. *New Engl J Med* **337**: 8–14.

# 10
# Systemic medications, IOP and management of open-angle glaucoma

General goals of medical management of glaucoma
Systemic medications and IOP
Topical ocular beta-blockers for control of IOP
Topical ocular adrenergics for control of IOP
Topical ocular carbonic anhydrase inhibitor
Topical ocular prostaglandin analogue
Topical ocular cholinergics (miotics)

## Introduction

Chronic open-angle glaucoma results from pathological changes in the optic disc and radiating nerve fibres, such that a discrete or more general change in the visual field develops. It is a progressive condition, usually developing over years. The changes develop as a result of both excessive fluid pressure (elevated intraocular pressure) and an imbalance in blood perfusion which may or may not be intimately related to the elevated IOP.

The measured IOP can simply be considered as reflecting the balance between the net fluid input into the eye via the ciliary epithelium compared with the net fluid exit from the eye via the trabecular meshwork and the uveoscleral pathway (Figure 10.1). This chapter will not address the complexity of the regulation of inflow and outflow of fluid from the eye but rather the clinical consequences of drug actions to alter IOP. The development of open-angle glaucoma can thus be associated with chronic ocular hypertension (i.e. primary open-angle glaucoma or simple glaucoma) or not (i.e. normal tension glaucoma or low-tension glaucoma). The elevation in

IOP without clinically significant changes in fundus appearance or the visual fields will generally be referred to as ocular hypertension (OHT) or the patients will be considered 'glaucoma suspects'.

All of these patients may be started on medical therapy which combines assessments of the appearance of the fundus, the IOP status and the dynamics of the visual field, with the use of drugs. While differences of opinion may emerge from time to time, strategies for medical management of open-angle glaucoma are still based on assessment of IOP, although the end-point for what would be considered as a satisfactory control of intraocular pressure will also be determined by consideration of fundus appearance and the state of the visual fields.

Periodic elevation in IOP (e.g. to a daily average pressure of 25 mmHg with a range of ±5 mmHg) is considered a risk factor for developing glaucoma. For these eyes and those with disc and field changes, medical therapy is still largely directed towards keeping daily average IOP closer to 18 mmHg than 25 mmHg (for example). There are no absolute values that can be given for a prescriptive strategy for medical

management of open-angle glaucoma. Current opinion is that tonometry measures can be influenced by central corneal thickness (CCT), with slightly higher IOP more likely to be recorded in patients with higher CCT values and *vice versa*.[1]

In terms of the goals of medical management, if a net reduction of 25% in the average daily IOP, achieved with topical medications, is found over many weeks or months to be associated with a stable fundus appearance and visual field then this would be considered as adequate, and perhaps the dosing could even be reduced to minimise the risk of adverse effects.

If further deterioration in the disc appearance and the visual field is still occurring, then the medical management needs to be more aggressive in the hope of achieving larger net reductions in IOP, e.g. by 30%, 35% or even 40%. By current medical strategies, larger changes cannot be achieved on a chronic basis and surgical intervention is needed.

The medical management of open-angle glaucoma is not a lightly undertaken activity for, once started, the therapies generally need to be continued. The key issue

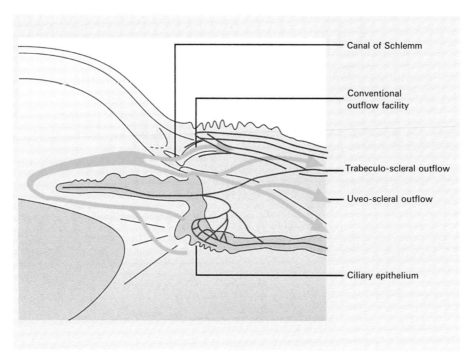

**Figure 10.1**
*Schematic illustration of the sites of action of antiglaucoma drugs.*

is whether the medication strategy adopted is effective at keeping IOP or vision stable, or both.[2] Equally important, especially by modern strategies, is how well the patient is able to achieve effective dosing (i.e. compliance with a medication regimen) and how well the patient tolerates the use of medications (i.e. that there is a relative freedom from adverse drug reactions).[2,3]

A non-compliant patient with open-angle glaucoma is less likely to be effectively managed, and a patient who develops even moderate ADRs from his or her glaucoma medications is less likely to be compliant.

All patients considered eligible for medical management of their open-angle glaucoma need to be carefully screened before starting medications to minimise the chance of severe systemic ADRs; these should generally be considered preventable provided patient screening and follow-up is comprehensive (see later).

Before deciding to use medications to manage open-angle glaucoma, several factors need to be considered. The availability of full eye examination beyond fundus assessment and tonometry is important, with at least some idea of the magnitude of the diurnal changes in IOP as well as when peak IOP occurs. Secondly, automated

perimetry (or a chosen equivalent) should have been performed on at least three independent visits separated by 1–2 months to confirm the visual field changes. The fundus appearance and the visual field changes should be consistent. A glaucoma suspect can thus expect to make several visits to a specialist (usually an ophthalmologist) before medications are prescribed.

When medications are prescribed, certain issues need to be considered. These relate to the risk of ADRs, concurrent medications and other diseases the patient may have, the planned intensity of medication use and the availability of long-term monitoring. The repeated use of eyedrops for glaucoma can have substantial adverse effects on autonomic function and so knowledge of all of a patient's medications is essential for prescribing 'anti-glaucoma' drugs.

Such ADRs may only become apparent during the routine monitoring of a glaucoma patient on medications. All patients with airways disease or cardiovascular disease should be carefully reviewed. Patients with long-standing diseases such as kidney failure, diabetes, high blood pressure or depression are less likely to show predictable responses to their anti-

glaucoma medications and more likely to show ADRs.

The magnitude of the IOP reduction that would be appropriate for a particular patient needs to be considered. Patients from ethnic groups with very darkly pigmented irides tend to be affected with open-angle glaucoma more often. This is important since the efficacy of all topical anti-glaucoma drugs is often less in these groups, and they are more likely to need multiple medications.

The goal of monitoring glaucoma patients on medications is to ensure freedom from ADRs and promote compliance with medication use, as well as to limit the chance of (rapid) deterioration in the visual fields. Patients need to be carefully checked for ADRs, and these are different for each type of glaucoma medication.

Patients also need to be instructed on the importance of taking every dose. Reminders and encouragements may be needed at regular intervals. Many months or years are generally required before definite improvements in the visual field can be expected and many patients will not show improvement, but just remain stable.

## Systemic medications and IOP

The medical management of open-angle glaucoma requires routine tonometry and its interpretation can only be useful if systemic medications are taken into account. A wide range of systemic medications can directly or indirectly change IOP. Medications may adversely affect IOP (i.e. increase IOP or the diurnal fluctuations in IOP) or change IOP such that the reliability of routine measurements is questionable (i.e. reduces IOP such that the patient is considered to be adequately controlled when they are not).

On the latter point, there is little evidence that systemic medications have any long-term beneficial effect in open-angle glaucoma, with the notable exception of carbonic anhydrase inhibitors (see later).

Many systemic medications can increase IOP from normally expected values, but there is no obvious consensus on this. The literature is littered with case reports associating the use of systemic medications with an increased IOP, but the regulatory agencies have adopted a range of guidelines.

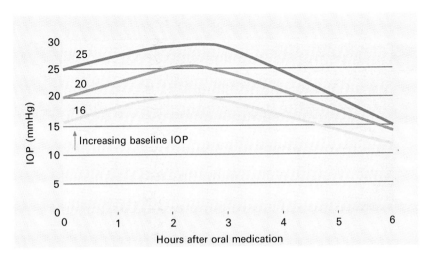

**Figure 10.2**
*Types of ocular hypertensive effects associated with use of systemic medications.*

Pharmaceutical directories (see Chapter 1) may include statements such as C/I (contraindications) for glaucoma or narrow-angle glaucoma, or even a personal or family history of narrow-angle glaucoma for use of these medications. Some guidelines are less prescriptive and state S/P (specific precautions) for glaucoma or narrow-angle glaucoma or increased IOP. All of these should be noted and it is also logical to take details of any medication for which listed ADRs include mydriasis and/or reduced accommodation even if there is no S/P note for narrow-angle glaucoma.

To review all of these differences in guidelines with respect to published reports is beyond the scope of this chapter. However, in the section below, a safety-first strategy is adopted to highlight patients for whom a little extra attention should be given in reviewing their medications, their glaucoma and possible glaucoma therapies. It should also be noted that even within a group of drugs with the same pharmacological mechanism, the absence of a specific precautionary note should not necessarily be taken as an indication that there is no risk of ocular hypertension developing.

In most cases, any IOP increase will be uneventful, other than there being a chance that slightly higher IOP values will be measured (Figure 10.2). The overall effects on IOP are usually small to modest, but it is important to note that such increases in intraocular pressure, if sustained, may be considered too much for some patients who already have elevated IOP values.

Equally importantly, the use of these medications could counteract the hypotensive effects of a patient's 'anti-glaucoma' medications. In rare cases, these systemic medications can precipitate angle-closure, with large increases in IOP developing (see Chapter 7).[4] Such medications are therefore C/I in patients with known narrow angles or pre-existing narrow-angle glaucoma, but many can still be used cautiously in patients with open-angle glaucoma.

The mechanisms by which IOP can be elevated are poorly defined. The medications range from 'drugs' used on a daily basis by millions with minimal risks, to those where some additional monitoring would be prudent to reduce risk, to those where, if possible, their use should be limited in open-angle glaucoma patients.

For example, there are still some who would advocate that the use of coffee and other caffeine-containing products should be monitored because they can cause small increases in IOP or alter ocular perfusion.[5,6] Similarly, the widely used oral histamine $H_1$-blocking drugs can increase IOP[7] and therefore there is a S/P for glaucoma for the older drugs in this class (e.g. chlorpheniramine, bromopheniramine, azatadine, mequitazine, promethazine or cyproheptadine) while it is absent for newer antihistamines (e.g. cetirizine, azelastine, acrivastine and mizolastine).

High doses of any systemic corticosteroids can increase IOP, sometimes substantially.[8,9] With progressive tapering of therapy to lower doses (perhaps even to

ultimate discontinuation), the IOP should return to normal levels (see Chapter 9). Commoner examples include oral or topical (skin) hydrocortisone and oral prednisolone, but inhaled or nasal corticosteroids such as beclomethasone or fluticasone should not be overlooked, especially in geriatric or paediatric patients.

Other drugs for which elevated IOP is a recognised ADR are the wide range of drugs with atropine-like (anticholinergic) actions. Here the risk is more for angle-closure developing but, as noted above, the recommendations for use in patients with glaucoma are variable; cautious use is probably possible in many patients.

Examples range from antinausea drugs sold as Pharmacy medicines (e.g. cyclizine, dimenhydrinate, and meclozine), drugs used to control nausea or protracted allergies (e.g. promethazine), special anti-asthma drugs such as ipratropium, special anti-arrhythmia drugs, for instance disopyramide, and antiparkinson's drugs including benzhexol, benztropine, biperiden and levodopa/carbidopa.

Other atropine-like drugs are used for alimentary tract disorders (e.g. hyoscine, dicyclomine), for urinary frequency control (e.g. propantheline, flavoxate, oxybutinin, or tolterodine) or to control nausea (e.g. hyoscine in P medicines or POM transdermal patches).

However, confusion can easily arise when considering medications for depression and anxiety and stress-related conditions such as migraine.[10,11] The anticholinergic side-effects are well known for a wide range of neuroactive drugs (see Chapter 3 for mechanisms) and include the tricyclic antidepressants (e.g. amitriptyline, trimipramine), tetracyclic antidepressants (eg maprotiline, mianserin), and some of the phenothiazine antipsychotics (e.g. chlorpromazine, thioridazine).

Benzodiazepine anxiolytics (e.g. diazepam, nitrazepam) are not known for any significant adverse effects on IOP. However, other antidepressants with indirect-adrenergic or indirect adrenergic/serotoninergic effects (see Chapter 3) are also widely used. These include:

- The monoamine oxidase (MAO) inhibitors such as phenelzine
- Reversible inhibitors of monoamine oxidase A (RIMAs) such as moclobemide
- Noradrenaline reuptake inhibitors (NARIs), e.g. reboxetine

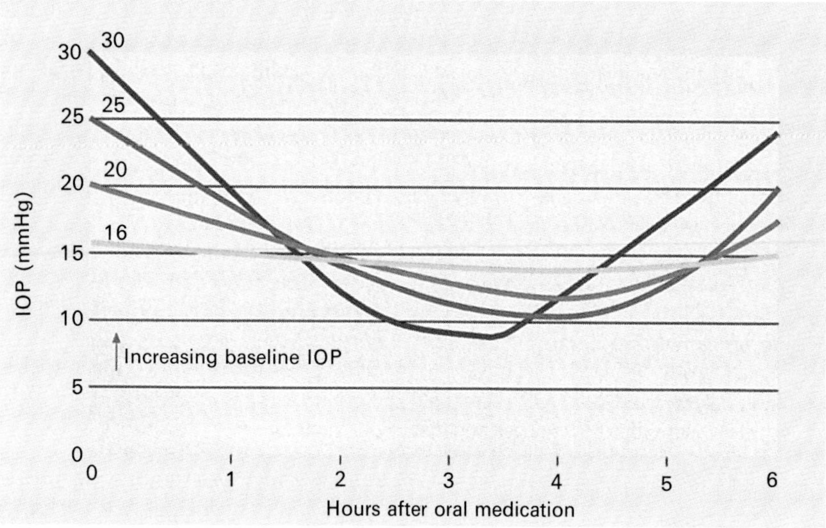

**Figure 10.3**
*Types of ocular hypotensive effects associated with use of systematic medications.*

- Noradrenaline and specific serotonin antidepressants (NaSSAs), e.g. mirtazapine
- Serotonin-noradrenaline reuptake inhibitors (SNRIs) such as venlafaxine
- Selective serotonin reuptake inhibitors (SSRIs) such as fluoxetine and paroxetine.

Some have anticholinergic effects (e.g. reboxetine) while others are not recognised for such an effect yet can still in rare cases cause angle-closure (see Chapter 7). For these adrenergic antiglaucoma medications, attention to observing contraindications for their use is more important than being concerned about angle-closure and/or ocular hypertension developing.

An equally large array of systemic medications can reduce IOP. There is unlikely to be any note about this in pharmaceutical directories because it is not considered an ADR. However, such changes in IOP may yield false results in screening or monitoring glaucoma patients. In most cases the changes can be expected only during a discrete period 1–4 hours after the medications were taken (Figure 10.3).

A slightly lower than normal IOP (for that patient) could be measured and this cycle will be repeated each time a patient takes the medication that affects the IOP.

The reductions in IOP may only be a few mmHg in normal patients, but reductions of 10 to 15 mmHg can occur in patients with ocular hypertension (Figure 10.3).

Drugs that most widely could reduce IOP are those that are used to lower blood pressure, with a 10 mmHg decrease in systolic pressure resulting in a 1–2 mmHg decrease in IOP.[10,12] Examples include beta-adrenergic-blocking drugs (e.g. propranolol), diuretics (e.g. acetazolamide, frusemide, hydrochlorothiazide, triamterene), vasodilators (e.g. clonidine, methyldopa or guanethidine, hydralazine), and drugs for congestive heart failure (e.g. digoxin).

Alcohol consumption, especially above the legal limit, can also reduce IOP, but there is insufficient evidence to indicate whether alcoholics will generally have a lower-than-expected IOP. Some ocular hypotensive effects are associated with the use of oral antidiabetic drugs (e.g. chlorpropamide) and more a reflection of the inadequacy of glycaemic control.

Bearing in mind that IOP commonly shows cyclical (diurnal) changes and that a wide range of systemic medications may slightly alter IOP, the medical management of glaucoma can be approached. The overall goal in the use of all current medications is to reduce IOP.

## Topical ocular beta-blockers for control of IOP

Topical ocular beta-blockers such as timolol are the most popular current medical therapies for open-angle glaucoma simply because they work and because the visual and systemic side-effects are generally minimal compared with other antiglaucoma medications.[12] However, the minimal risk of systemic side-effects can only be realised if care is taken not to use these drugs on the wrong patients.[3]

The early enthusiasm[13] that timolol eyedrops were 'effective in reducing the intraocular pressure in a glaucoma patient without producing any serious side-effects' has been proven to be grossly incorrect. A wide range of systemic side-effects can develop[3,14,15] as a result of absorption of timolol into the conjunctiva and through to the systemic circulation (see Chapter 2).[3,16] Therefore, the listed C/I for use of all topical beta-adrenergic blockers for glaucoma include a history of bronchospasm, bronchial asthma or any chronic airways disease or pulmonary obstruction.

All these ophthalmic beta-blockers are also contraindicated in patients with sinus bradycardia or any serious cardiac conduction-block, as well as patients with recent history of congestive heart failure, severe shock or trauma. Warnings for the use of topical ocular beta-blockers note that they should be used with caution (and perhaps not at all) if reasonable alternatives are available in patients with labile diabetes, who are pregnant or who are taking certain medications for high blood pressure and angina (e.g. verapamil), or vasodilators for high blood pressure (e.g. clonidine and guanethidine). For patients with mild airways disease, a cardioselective topical ophthalmic beta-blocker (betaxolol) may be used (see below).

Special precautions for the use of topical ocular beta-blockers note that they should be used cautiously, or avoided, if a patient has medication with systemic beta-blockers (for high blood pressure, arrhythmias or migraine). For any glaucoma patient with blood pressure problems, monitoring pulse rate and blood pressure should be a constituent part of every eye examination.

Ocular beta-blockers are generally for patients whose daily average IOP is less than 30 mmHg, i.e. closer to 25 mmHg. Their mechanism of action primarily involves a reduction in the net rate of aqueous humour secretion, with little effect on outflow facility. No change in the pupil diameter is expected with the use of topical ocular beta-blockers.

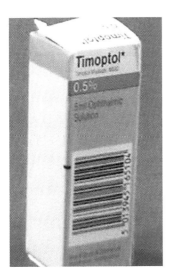

**Figure 10.4**
*Timolol 0.5% eyedrops.*

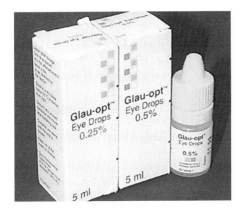

**Figure 10.5**
*Timolol 0.25% or 0.5% eyedrops, generic.*

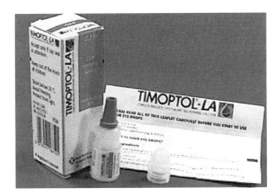

**Figure 10.6**
*Timolol 0.25% ophthalmic gel.*

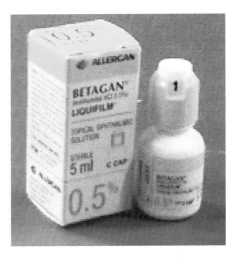

**Figure 10.7**
*Levobunolol 0.5% eyedrops.*

## Timolol

The first ocular beta-blocker was timolol eyedrops.[17] Timolol is a non-selective beta-blocker with a high potential for causing bronchopulmonary ADRs. Products available include both the initial product, POM Timoptol (Figure 10.4) and generic equivalents, e.g. POM Glau-Opt, (Figure 10.5) or other generics simply labelled as Timolol Eye Drops. All are available at two concentrations, 0.25% and 0.5%, and dispensed in 5 ml bottles.

Unit-dose and preservative-free Timoptol is still listed as available for special cases (see below), while other unit dose preparations have been available.

For the most part, dosing with timolol eyedrops should be twice-daily (*bds*) and generally with both eyes treated. Initially, the lower concentration of 0.25% may be used, moving to the higher concentration if further control is needed and providing the patient is free of systemic ADRs. As a result of the risk of systemic ADRs, there is no indication for more frequent use of timolol eyedrops for open-angle glaucoma. A few patients may be managed on a once-daily regimen.

Beyond an expected transient stinging or irritation on instillation, some patients may develop local intolerance to ophthalmic beta-blockers and need to be switched to a preservative-free product. Such patients may include those with dry eye or other ocular surface diseases (see below).

For selected patients, a special timolol eye 'gel' (POM Timoptol-LA, Figure 10.6) may be used, usually on a once-daily regimen, and is preferable to the use of eyedrops for patients on once-daily treatment. The eyedrop is very viscous and forms a gel on mixing with the tear film.[18]

## Levobunolol

The second ophthalmic beta-blocker is levobunolol and is used at the 0.5% concentration as eyedrops available as POM Betagan in 5 ml bottles (Figure 10.7) and unit-dose preparations (not illustrated). As with timolol, the recommended dosing is usually twice-daily. The special C-CAP changes from number 1 to number 2 and back to 1 as the bottle is cyclically opened for twice-daily dosing. A generic levobunolol 0.5% may also be available (without the C-CAP).

Levobunolol is a non-selective beta-blocker with a high potential for causing bronchopulmonary ADRs. Its long-term efficacy is generally equivalent to timolol 0.5% eyedrops.[19] POM Betagan contains bisulphites, which can precipitate substantial allergic reactions.

## Betaxolol

The third ophthalmic beta-blocker is betaxolol. This is now generally used as a special microfine 0.25% suspension (POM Betoptic Suspension) available in a 5 ml bottle (Figure 10.8). As with timolol, the recommended dosing is usually twice-daily.[20]

Betaxolol is classified as a cardioselective beta-adrenergic blocker, i.e. more selectively acts on cardiac $beta_1$-receptors rather than equally on cardiac $beta_2$-receptors and bronchial $beta_2$-receptors. It was introduced in the mid-1980s as the drug to overcome the limitations in the use of timolol and levobunolol. The repeated use of betaxolol 0.5% eyedrops can still

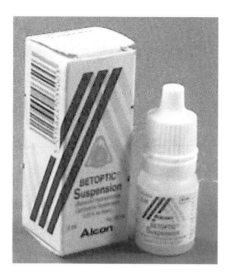

**Figure 10.8**
*Betaxolol 0.25% ophthalmic suspension.*

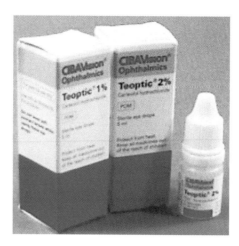

**Figure 10.9**
*Carteolol 1% and 2% eyedrops.*

cause life-threatening bronchospasm in asthmatic patients. The CSM continues to advise careful monitoring, and that it should only be used in patients with airways disease if other medical options are not available.

The older betaxolol 0.5% eyedrops (POM Betoptic) are still available and their efficacy is considered equivalent to the 0.25% betaxolol suspension. However, the second characteristic of this beta-blocker product is the special formulation which is designed to reduce even further the risk of systemic side-effects.

The suspension is such that, on mixing with the tear film, the drug is slowly released to provide extended delivery.[21]

With the use of a microfine suspension, the rate of drainage of the suspension down the nasolacrimal duct to the systemic circulation (see Chapter 2) can be expected to be slower and so the risk of acute systemic changes is less. Overall, therefore, the risk of systemic ADRs with Betoptic-S can be expected to be lower than other ocular beta-blockers.

However, patient intolerance of the special formulation could still be an issue, and betaxolol in itself may not have adequate ocular hypotensive effects compared with timolol or levobunolol.[22]

### Carteolol
A fourth ocular beta-blocker is carteolol. This is used at the 1% or 2% concentration and is available as POM Teoptic in 5 ml bottles (Figure 10.9). As with timolol, the recommended dosing is usually twice-daily, and the option is also for use of a lower concentration for initial management and increasing it later – carteolol 1% is considered equivalent to timolol 0.25%.

Carteolol is a non-selective beta-adrenergic blocker like timolol and levobunolol, but as a result of its chemical structure also has 'intrinsic sympathomimetic activity' or ISA. This agonist effect is designed to offset some of the systemic blocking effects, as well as have ocular adrenergic effects (see below). Any reduction in the risk of systemic bronchopulmonary ADRs must be considered as advantageous.

The dual action on IOP should improve its control, although clinical studies do not indicate that carteolol eyedrops are any more effective than timolol.[23]

### Metipranolol
The other ocular beta-blocker marketed in the UK is metipranolol. It is a non-selective beta-blocker with a high potential for causing bronchopulmonary adverse effects[24] and is available as POM Minims Metipranolol. Its use is limited because it can cause granulomatous or non-granulomatous uveitis.[25,26]

Manufacturers' guidelines on the use of all topical ocular beta-blockers include notes to the effect that therapy should be discontinued if a severe dry eye or other inflammatory condition develops. As a result, metipranolol is unlikely to be used much at this time in the UK, especially because other unit-dose products are available. The warnings for use of topical ocular beta-blockers in patients with dry eyes is

more prominent for carteolol-containing products, but it is uncertain if this is a formulation-related issue or a unique toxic effect (leading to conjunctivitis and keratitis) that results from the chemical properties of carteolol.

Carteolol has another special chemical property called MSA (membrane-stabilising activity) which it also shares with levobunolol and metipranolol, and perhaps timolol.[12] This property has no obvious impact on the clinical efficacy of topical ocular beta-blockers but differences in MSA could be the reason why some beta-blockers (e.g. carteolol) may be more likely to produce epithelial changes that are similar to those produced by topical ocular anaesthetics. Indeed, it can be expected that some patients on long-term therapy with any of the topical ocular beta-blockers may develop some degree of corneal hypothaesia.[12]

In most cases, providing systemic effects do not develop, long-term ocular tolerance to ophthalmic beta-blockers is good and the patient can be maintained on the beta-blocker therapy (at the appropriate dose and regimen) for at least one and maybe 2 years without need for change.

Initially, the patients will generally be seen at 2 weeks and 1 month to ensure that the IOP reduction has been achieved. The prescribed therapy (if adequate) will produce the required lowering of IOP within a week in most patients, but some fail to show an adequate response and need early dosage adjustment. These initial visits are also important to identify any ADRs.

Longer-term follow-up/check-up generally requires visits every 2 or 3 months during the first year of therapy, with new pharmaceutical prescriptions being written at each visit.

After this time period, visits need to be regularly spaced, but depend on individual patient responses to the medication (providing there are no marked changes in visual fields and no ADRs).

For some patients even maximum therapy with beta-blockers will not be adequate, while others can become refractory to this therapy rather quickly (sometimes referred to as 'escape' phenomena). Various supplemental options are available that could include the addition of adrenergic eyedrops, miotics, or topical or oral carbonic anhydrase inhibitors (see below).

## Topical adrenergics for control of IOP

Not all glaucoma patients or glaucoma suspects can be treated with topical ocular beta-blockers. Their use may be contraindicated, the patient might develop intolerance or there may be a concern that he or she is at risk for, or has developed, other side-effects such as depression, loss of libido, etc.[3,14] Other starting medications are thus needed.

Before the introduction of timolol, adrenaline eyedrops (and/or the use of miotics) were common place. Many years of clinical use of adrenaline eyedrops has established that such adrenergic therapy is 'safer' than ophthalmic beta-adrenergic blocker therapy, and there are essentially none of the contraindications or warnings of the type needed for use of beta-blockers in patients with pulmonary disease or dysfunction.

Cases of systemic sympathomimetic responses to adrenergic eyedrops were uncommon, but there are some limits to the use of adrenergics, especially with current guidelines. The potential for sympathomimetic effects cannot be ignored and so ophthalmic adrenergic drugs for glaucoma control should be limited (S/P) in patients with severe cardiovascular disease, stroke and severe peripheral circulatory problems (e.g. Raynaud's syndrome).

Their use should also be limited or avoided in patients using a wide range of medications for severe hypertension (e.g. clonidine and guanethidine), or severe cardiovascular conditions (e.g. digoxin). For any ophthalmic adrenergic therapy, concurrent medication with any systemic sympathomimetics is not recommended, and so should be limited or avoided in patients medicated with MAO inhibitors and any other 'antidepressants affecting noradrenergic transmission', i.e. RIMAs, NARIs, NaSSAs, SNRIs, tricyclic antidepressants and tetracyclic antidepressants (see above and Chapter 3).

Several adrenergic options are listed for the UK, but only two are used regularly, i.e. brimonidine and dipivefrin. The others are either still available for patients adequately controlled with them (e.g. adrenaline or guanethidine eyedrops) or are only indicated in the UK for short-term use prior to surgery (e.g. apraclonidine).

### Brimonidine

The current most widely prescribed adrenergic for glaucoma is likely to be brimonidine, available as 0.2% eyedrops as POM Alphagan in a 5 ml bottle with C-CAP (see Chapter 4). It is the modern substitute for adrenaline eyedrops.[27] POM Alphagan is for twice-daily usage in the UK, and generally for patients with average IOPs of less than 30 mmHg.

Modest reductions in IOP (i.e. 15–20 per cent) can be expected within a week and perhaps slightly greater increases over several weeks, up to 25 per cent reductions. In other words, POM Alphagan can be expected to show a clinical efficacy similar to the use of adrenaline 2% eyedrops, but generally slightly less than timolol 0.5%. The main hypotensive mechanism is by decreased aqueous production via alpha$_2$-adrenergic receptors that are stimulated by brimonidine; some increase in uveoscleral outflow is expected.

Compared with chronic use of adrenaline eyedrops (see below), brimonidine eyedrops are considered to have a lesser potential for irritating the conjunctiva, but follicular conjunctivitis can still develop. POM Alphagan eyedrops also contain bisulphites. Patient follow-up generally needs to be less rigorous compared with ophthalmic beta-blockers, but visits at one and three months and then every three to six months is not unusual.

The minimum of the six-monthly check is to assess for possible irritative reactions to the conjunctiva. Should the control of IOP with brimonidine 0.2% eyedrops be inadequate, it probably can be supplemented with miotics (see below under dipivefrin) but there are limited clinical data at this time for such dual therapy.

### Dipivefrin

A second ophthalmic adrenergic therapy option is with dipivefrin, which is an ester derivative of adrenaline (epinephrine), i.e. dipivalyl epinephrine.[28] It is available at the 0.1% concentration as POM Propine (Figure 10.10) in a 5 ml bottle with C-CAP. Generic dipivefrin eyedrops are also available.

Dipivefrin was introduced in the 1980s as an alternative to adrenaline, and is generally for twice-daily use (not *qd* and is rarely used *tds*). When used for patients with average IOPs of less than 30 mmHg, modest reductions in IOP (i.e. 10–15 per cent) can be expected within a week and

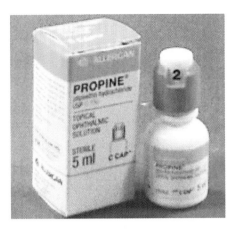

**Figure 10.10**
*Dipivefrin 0.1% eyedrops.*

perhaps slightly greater increases over several weeks, i.e. up to 20 per cent.

Dipivefrin, as a pro-drug, has greater corneal penetration than epinephrine and is rapidly biotransformed (metabolised) to epinephrine by the cornea.

As a pro-drug it only needs to be administered at low doses to achieve an ocular hypotensive effect equivalent to adrenaline 1% or 2%, although clinical data indicates that it is unlikely to actually achieve this full effect in the long term. However, with the use of low concentrations, the overall chance of development of local ocular side-effects (irritation, lacrimation, rebound hyperaemia, etc.) is less than with adrenaline. POM Propine formulations contain bisulphites.

The use of dipivefrin 0.1% eyedrops can also cause slight mydriasis and should be used with caution until the true nature of the glaucoma has been firmly established.

Patient follow-up is generally as for those receiving therapy with brimonidine eyedrops.

If IOP control is inadequate, the therapy can be supplemented by keeping the patient on dipivefrin *bds* and adding pilocarpine eyedrops at an appropriate concentration *bds* or *tds*. The dipivefrin eyedrops should be instilled 10 minutes after the pilocarpine. The starting pilocarpine concentration can usually be low (e.g. 0.5% or 1% and later there is then the option to increase the pilocarpine concentration to 2%, 3%, or 4%).

Alternatively, the dipivefrin eyedrops can be maintained *bds* and topical or oral carbonic anhydrase inhibitors added (see later).

### Adrenaline

Epinephrine (adrenaline) eyedrops are still available as POM Simplene (7.5 ml bottle, 0.5% and 1% eyedrops; see Chapter 4) and POM Eppy (7.5 ml bottles, 1% eyedrops). Epinephrine eyedrops will generally be used on patients with IOPs below 30 mmHg, and are generally used *bds* (and perhaps *tds*) with the option to use the lower concentration as starting therapy.[29,30]

Moderate reductions in IOP (15–20 per cent) can be expected within a week and perhaps slightly greater increases over several weeks, i.e. up to 30 per cent. Epinephrine ophthalmic solutions can contain low concentrations of acetylcysteine as a stabiliser. Epinephrine eyedrops can cause mydriasis (see dipivefrin).

Perhaps the greatest limit to the use of adrenaline eyedrops is the risk of developing local ocular side-effects such as irritation, lacrimation, rebound hyperaemia, etc. Furthermore, chronic use of epinephrine eyedrops can cause a condition called ocular 'melanosis', also referred to as 'adrenochrome' deposits, or adrenomelanoses.[31] It is probably for this reason, and because it is an avoidable ADR (as other adrenergics such as brimonidine or dipivefrin are available), that these eyedrops are unlikely to be newly prescribed .

The deposits can be black or very dark brown and appear on the conjunctiva, the conjunctival crypts, and puncta. They can also look like black mascara in early stages and can be irritating.

Where appropriate, epinephrine eyedrop therapy can be supplemented with miotics or topical or oral carbonic anhydrase inhibitors could be added (see section on dipivefrin above).

Adrenaline is also still available in combination with guanethidine in a unique product, POM Ganda Eye Drops (7.5 ml bottles). The use of POM Ganda is principally for patients already established on this therapy. Two combinations are available known as '1 + 0.2' (which is guanethidine 1% with adrenaline 0.2%) and '3 + 0.5' (which is guanethidine 3% with adrenaline 0.5%).[32]

### Apraclonidine

This is the last ophthalmic adrenergic for glaucoma (i.e. as a 0.5% solution as POM Iopidine). Its original indication was to ocular hypertension developing after laser surgery to the eye but it is also now approved for short-term management for glaucoma before surgery.[33]

## Topical carbonic anhydrase inhibitor

Dorzolamide was introduced in 1995 as a special topical carbonic anhydrase inhibitor (CAI) 2% solution as POM Trusopt (5 ml bottle). A second topical CAI, brinzolamide 1% ophthalmic suspension (POM Azopt, 5 ml bottle) was introduced in 2000. Both are only indicated for use in the UK for management of open-angle glaucoma unresponsive to beta-blockers or for patients for whom beta-blocker therapy is contraindicated. These drugs inhibit the carbonic anhydrase-dependent aqueous humour secretion and so lower IOP.[34]

POM Trusopt should generally be used *tds*, but can be used *bds* as a supplementary therapy to beta-blockers, adrenergics or miotics. To facilitate such dual therapy, a dorzolamide 2%–timolol 0.5% combination eyedrop (POM Cosopt) is available for *bds* use. When used as a monotherapy, the dosing really needs to be *tds* and even then the expected ocular hypotensive effects are unlikely to even approach those achieved with timolol 0.5% *bds*.

Based on data available, it is likely that topical CAIs will only be useful in patients with average IOPs less than 30 mmHg, and perhaps somewhat less than this. There are other limits to the use of topical CAIs in that their use is contraindicated in patients with severe kidney diseases of any type, and they should be used cautiously in patients with known sulphonamide drug allergy, or severe hepatic disease.

The use of dorzolamide or brinzolamide eyedrops is not expected to produce substantial systemic ADRs of the type that limit the use of topical ocular beta-blockers (although consideration of such systemic side-effects is of paramount importance if a combination therapy of dorzolamide with timolol (POM Cosopt) is used). Their use may be unpleasant for some in that they tend to leave a bitter taste in the mouth but otherwise appear to be well tolerated compared with topical beta-blockers.

An issue that has been raised is whether the intensive use of a topical CAI would compromise the corneal endothelial function.[34–36] To date, significant problems have not been reported[34,35] which indicates that the role of carbonic anhydrase in endothelial function is minimal.[36] However, it remains to be established whether certain patients should be screened for endothelial status before and during topical CAI therapy.[34,35]

All topical antiglaucoma therapies can be supplemented on a short-term basis with an oral CAI, acetazolamide. Acetazolamide enters the eye via the ciliary circulation to inhibit carbonic anhydrase-dependent aqueous humour secretion. While drugs of this type were once widely used, the high incidence of systemic ADRs limits their use nowadays.

Oral acetazolamide is generally prescribed as sustained-release capsules (250 mg, POM Diamox SR) as an adjunct to the topical glaucoma medications and usually on a daily (or *bds*) regimen, e.g. as a night-time supplement to topical therapies.[37,38] A range of general adverse effects (tiredness, malaise, etc) can develop following oral acetazolamide therapy.[37] As a diuretic, oral acetazolamide can lower blood pressure and reduce blood potassium iron ($K^+$) levels (hypokalaemia) so blood electrolytes data should be regularly available, and $K^+$ supplements considered.

Oral acetazolamide should not be used (as general antiglaucoma drugs) in patients with severe kidney dysfunction (who will likely have electrolyte imbalances), and should also be avoided in patients with adrenal insufficiencies or hepatic dysfunction.

Oral acetazolamide should be used cautiously in patients using high doses of certain NSAIDs (e.g. acetylsalicylic acid or other salicylates),[39] systemic corticosteroids (e.g. prednisolone and perhaps other steroids in general), and anticoagulants (e.g. heparin). These drugs can also cause a unique type of allergic or hypersensitivity reaction which, in the extreme, can cause severe rashes and/or a general blood dyscrasia.

Therefore, as well as checking for allergy to carbonic anhydrase inhibitors, a check needs to be made for potential allergy to related compounds such as sulphonamide anti-infective drugs and some oral antidiabetes drugs, the sulphonylureas (e.g. chlorpropamide).

The sulphonamides may also be referred to as folic acid antagonists because this is the mechanism of their antibacterial action (see Chapter 8), and sulphonylureas as oral hypoglycaemic drugs because they promote insulin release and thus lower the blood sugar levels.

## Topical prostaglandin analogue

A new option for glaucoma therapy was introduced in 1997. Latanoprost is a topical prostaglandin analogue, specifically an ester of prostaglandin $F_{2\alpha}$ and is available as POM Xalatan 0.005% eyedrops (2.5 ml special bottle; see Chapter 4). Latanoprost is a prostaglandin pro-drug indicated for once-daily use in the UK, preferably in the evening, but only for uncomplicated cases of open-angle glaucoma.[40]

Data from clinical trials indicate that even once-daily dosing with latanoprost 0.005% eyedrops should provide equivalent hypotensive effects to timolol 0.5% *bds*.

Latanoprost appears uniquely to reduce IOP by increasing the uveoscleral (as opposed to trabeculoscleral) outflow from the eye. As a result, latanoprost is not generally indicated for concurrent use with miotics, but adjunct therapy with beta-blockers, dipivefrin, topical or oral carbonic anhydrase inhibitors appears to be effective.

However, this novel option is not without its problems and it is likely that long-term use will reveal a number of significant limitations.[40–42] At this time, patients on latanoprost therapy should be carefully monitored for conjunctival irritation (generally manifest as substantial hyperaemia) or iris changes (a drug-associated change in iris colour, or heterochromia, especially in those with hazel irides).

The conjunctival vasodilation and resultant irritation is an expected effect of a prostaglandin and it is unlikely to be any worse than that which can develop following chronic use of miotic (see below). However, there is further concern that latanoprost use may cause intraocular inflammation and unpublished guidelines suggest that this option for IOP control is not viable for aphakic patients or those with past history of ocular inflammation or macular disease. There is also concern that the chronic use of latanoprost eyedrops could also produce abnormalities of the eyelashes, including growth of a second row of eyelashes.

## Topical cholinergics (miotics)

Miotics formed the mainstay of glaucoma therapy for over 50 years, but are now only used as a starting medication on patients with average IOPs over 30 mmHg, or those who have very darkly pigmented eyes. Two options are available, namely pilocarpine as eyedrops or a gel, and carbachol eyedrops. Other special options include a pilocarpine insert (POM Ocusert Pilo)[43] and an indirect-acting cholinergic, echothiophate[44] now only available as eyedrops for hospital use.

The efficacy of miotics such as pilocarpine is very much related to ocular pigmentation, although concentrations of the drug are available (i.e. 4%) that allow one to largely overcome the pigmentation effects. Lower concentrations of pilocarpine (0.5% to 2%) are generally for use as supplements to beta-blocker or adrenergic therapies rather than for use as primary treatments.

The miotic therapy primarily produces a reduction in IOP by opening up the canal of Schlemm as a result of contracting the ciliary muscles and so increasing outflow facility. It has been periodically debated whether direct-acting cholinergics can also reduce slightly aqueous humour secretion. The miosis is not the actual cause of the increased trabeculoscleral outflow facility, but increased outflow is unlikely if an obvious miosis does not develop. The substantial miosis can reduce vision and produce artefacts in visual fields assessments.

Repeated use of miotics as long-term glaucoma therapy is to be avoided in any patient where miosis is undesirable, e.g. patients with a history of intraocular inflammation. Miotics will further dilate the blood vessels and put the patient at risk for iris bombé. Miotic therapy is generally not indicated for use in patients with lighter pigmented (blue) eyes because of the pronounced miosis that can accompany the hypotensive action of these drugs in lightly-pigmented eyes. The repeated use of pilocarpine (or other miotics) can lead to substantial visual acuity changes (due to pseudomyopia) in younger glaucoma patients. Pronounced ciliary body spasm may also accompany the initial use of these drugs, but an adaptive effect is usually seen within a week or so.

Miotic therapy also tends to be uncomfortable, and cosmetically unappealing (due to cholinergic vasodilation on the bulbar conjunctiva). Excessive lacrimation and even epiphora can also be present. There is renewed debate as to whether the use of cholinergic eyedrops should be considered a risk in either asthmatic patients or those with cardiac insufficiency; parasympathetic effects on the lungs and heart have been occasionally reported following the use of eyedrops containing carbachol.

Pilocarpine is available at the 0.5%, 1%, 2%, 3% and 4% concentrations as POM Isopto Carpine (10 ml bottles) and in a range of generic products (see Chapter 4). A 4% pilocarpine carbomer 934 gel formulation (POM Pilogel, 5 g tube) was introduced for the UK market in 1996. Carbachol comes at the 3% concentration as POM Isopto Carbachol (10 ml bottles).

Miotic therapy should be started *tds* or *qds* at a concentration commensurate with the ocular hypotensive effect required (with the ultimate goal of reducing the IOP to less than 20 mmHg); the miosis is substantially dependent upon the pilocarpine concentration and on ocular pigmentation.[45–47] The full effect does not have to be produced immediately, i.e. a patient can be started on a lower concentration such as 2% pilocarpine for a few weeks then shifted up to a higher concentration and with the option of using a pilocarpine 4% gel for overnight use (i.e. applied just before going to bed).[48]

As an alternative, the pilocarpine insert (POM Ocusert-Pilo) P-20 or P-40 may be tried, especially if a patient is having difficulty with eyedrop instillation, or maintaining a *qds* regimen.[43] These Ocusert devices deliver pilocarpine at a constant rate to the ocular surface with the P-20 releasing 20 µg/hour and the P-40 40 µg/hour. The patient requires careful instruction on how and when to insert and remove/replace the device and must be able to tolerate the insert (that can be likened to hard contact lens) as well as be sufficiently aware of it (in case it falls out). Generally, the device will be in place for 7 days before being replaced. The Ocusert inserts must be stored in a refrigerator.

## References

1 Doughty MJ, Zaman ML (2000) Human corneal thickness and its impact on intraocular pressure measures: a review and meta-analysis approach. *Surv Ophthalmol* **44**: 367–408.

2 Begg IS, Cottle RW (1988) Epidemiologic approach to open-angle glaucoma: I. Control of intraocular pressure. Report of the Canadian ocular adverse drug reaction registry program. *Can J Ophthalmol* **23**: 273–278.

3 Urtti A, Salminen L (1993) Minimizing systematic absorption of topically administered ophthalmic drugs. *Surv Ophthalmol* **37**: 435–456.

4 Doughty MJ (1997) Pupillary dilation. The standard for delivery of primary eye care. *Optometry Today* Nov 14, pp. 27–31.

5 Higginbotham EJ, Kilimanjaro HA, Wilensky JT *et al.* (1989) The effect of caffeine on intraocular pressure in glaucoma patients. *Ophthalmology* **96**: 624–626.

6 Lofti K, Grunwald JE (1991) The effect of caffeine on the human macular circulation. *Invest Ophthalmol Vis Sci* **32**: 3028–3032.

7 Cellini M, Profazio V, Barbaresi E (1982) Comportamento dell'oftalmotono dopo somministrazone orale di antihistaminica. *Ann Ottalmol Clin Oculist* **108**: 901–906.

8 Tripathi RC, Kirschner BS, Kipp M *et al.* (1992) Corticosteroid treatment for inflammatory bowel disease in pediatric patients increases intraocular pressure. *Gastroenterol* **102**: 1957–1961.

9 Opatowsky I, Feldman RM, Gross R, Feldman ST (1995) Intraocular pressure elevation associated with inhalation and nasal corticosteroids. *Ophthalmology* **102**: 177–179.

10 Doughty MJ, Lyle WM (1995) Medications used to prevent migraine headaches and their potential ocular adverse effects. *Optom Vis Sci* **72**: 879–891.

11 Doughty MJ (1999) The ocular side effects of CNS-acting drugs. *Optician* **218**: 17–26.

12 Doughty MJ, Lyle WM (1987) The development of beta-adrenergic blocking drugs for the management of primary open-angle glaucoma. *Can J Optom* **49**: 195–202.

13 Maino JH (1979) Timoptic: a new glaucoma medication. *Rev Optom* Feb. pp. 81–83.

14 Fraunfelder FT, Meyer SM (1987) Systemic side effects from ophthalmic timolol and their prevention. *J Ocular Pharmacol* **3**: 177–184.

15 Le Jeunne CL, Hugues FC, Duier JL *et al.* (1989) Bronchial and cardiovascular effects of ocular topical b-antagonists in asthmatic subjects: comparison of timolol, carteolol, and metipranolol. *J Clin Pharmacol* **29**: 97–101.

16 Vuori M-L, Kaila T (1995) Plasma kinetics and antagonist activity of topical ocular timolol in elderly patients. *Graefe's Arch Clin Exp Ophthalmol* **233**: 131–134.

17 Zimmerman TJ, Kaufman HE (1977) Timolol. A beta-adrenergic blocking agent for the treatment of glaucoma. *Arch Ophthalmol* **95**: 601–604.

18 Laurence J, Holder D, Vogel R *et al.* (1993) A double-masked, placebo-controlled evaluation of timolol in gel vehicle. *J Glaucoma* **2**: 177–181.

19 Levobunolol Study Group (1989) Levobunolol. A four-year study of efficacy and safety in glaucoma treatment. *Ophthalmology* **96**: 642–645.

20 Weinreb RN, Caldwell DR, Goode SM *et al.* (1990) A double-masked three month comparison between 0.25% betaxolol suspension and 0.5% betaxolol ophthalmic solution. *Am J Ophthalmol* **110**: 189–192.

21 Jani R, Gan O, Ali Y *et al.* (1994) Ion exchange resins for ophthalmic delivery. *J Ocular Pharmacol* **10**: 57–67.

22 Feghali JG, Kaufman PL, Radius RL *et al.* (1988) A comparison of betaxolol and timolol in opne angle glaucoma and ocular hypertension. *Acta Ophthalmol* **66**: 180–186.

23 Crisp P, Sorkin EM (1992) Ocular carteolol. A review of its pharmacological properties and therapeutic use in glaucoma and ocular hypertension. *Drugs Aging* **2**: 58–77.

24 Battershill PE, Sorkin EM (1988) Ocular metipranolol – a preliminary review of its pharmacodynamic and pharmacokinetic properties, and therapeutic efficacy in glaucoma and ocular hypertenson. *Drugs* **36**: 601–615.

25 Schultz JS, Hoenig JA, Chalres H (1993) Possible bilateral anterior uveitis secondary to metipranolol (Optipranolol) therapy. *Arch Ophthalmol* **111**: 1606–1607.

26 Akingbehin T, Villada JR, Walley T (1992) Metipranolol-induced adverse reactions. The rechallenge study. *Eye* **6**: 277–279.

27 Schuman JS (1996) Clinical experience with brimonidine 0.2% and timolol 0.5% in glaucoma and ocular hypertension. *Surv Ophthalmol* **41** (S-1): S27–S37.

28 Mandell AI, Stenz F, Kitabchi AE (1978) Dipivalyl epinephrine: a new pro-drug in the treatment of glaucoma. *Ophthalmology* **85**: 268–275.

29 Becker B, Morton WR (1966) Topical epinephrine in glaucoma suspects. *Am J Ophthalmol* **62**: 272–276.

30 Kass MA, Mandell AI, Goldberg I *et al.* (1979) Dipivefrin and epinephrine treatment of elevated intraocular pressure: a comparative study. *Arch Ophthalmol* **97**: 1865–1866.

31 Doughty MJ (1996) Diagnostic and therapeutic pharmaceutical agents for use in contact lens practice. In: *Clinical Contact Lens Practice* (Bennett ED, Weissman BA, eds). JB Lippincott, Philadelphia, USA Chapter 9, pp. 1–38.

32 Romano J, Patterson G (1979) Evaluation of a 5% guanethidine and 0.5% adrenaline mixture (Ganda 5.05) and of a 3% guanethidine and 0.5% adrenaline mixture (Ganda 3.05) in the treatment of glaucoma. *Br J Ophthalmol* **62**: 52–55.

33 Robin AL, Ritch R, Shin DH *et al.* (1995) Short-term efficacy of apraclonidine hydrochloride added to maximum-tolerated medical therapy for glaucoma. *Am J Ophthalmol* **120**: 423–432.

34 Balfour JA, Wilde MI (1997) Dorzolamide. A review of its pharmacology and therapeutic potential in the management of glaucoma and ocular hypertension. *Drugs Aging* **10**: 384–403.

35 Konowal A, Morrison JC, Brown SV *et al.* (1999) Irreversible corneal decompensation in patients treated with topical dorzolamide. *Am J Ohthalmol* **127**: 403–406.

36 Doughty MJ (1985) Prognosis for long-term topical carbonic anhydrase inhibitors and glaucoma management. *Topics Ocular Pharmacol Toxicol* **1**: 41–44.

37 Berson FG (1982) Carbonic anhydrase inhibitors of the eye – a review. *J Toxicol Cut Ocular Toxicol* **1**: 169–179.

38 Joyce PW, Mills KB (1990) Comparison of the effect of acetazolamide tablets and Sustets on diurnal intraocular pressure in patients with chronic simple glaucoma. *Br J Ophthalmol* **74**: 413–416.

39 Hazouard E, Grimbert M, Jonville-Berra A-P *et al.* (1999) Salicylisme et glaucoma: augmentation reciproque de la toxicite de l'acetazolamide et de l'acide acetyl salicylique. *J Fr Ophthalmol* **22**: 73–75.

40 Watson PG (1998) Latanoprost. Two years' experience of its use in the United Kingdom. *Ophthalmology* **105**: 82–87.

41 Wistrand PJ, Stjerschantz J, Olsson K (1997) The incidence and time-course of latanoprost-induced iridial pigmentation as a function of eye color. *Surv Ophthalmol* **41** (S-2): S129–S138.

42 Ayyala RS, Cruz DA, Margo CE *et al.* (1998) Cystoid macula edema associated with latanoprost in aphakic and pseudoaphakic eyes. *Am J Ophthalmol* **126**: 602–604.

43 Smith SE, Smith SA, Friedmann AI *et al.* (1979) Comparison of the pupillary, refractive and hypotensive effects of Ocusert-40 and pilocarpine eyedrops in the management of chronic simple glaucoma. *Br J Ophthalmol* **63**: 228–232.

44 Harris LS (1971) Dose-response analysis of echothiophate iodide. *Arch Ophthalmol* **86**: 502–511.

45 Harris LS, Gallin MA (1970) Dose-response analysis of pilocarpine-induced ocular hypotension. *Arch Ophthalmol* **84**: 605–608.

46 Harris LS, Gallin MA (1971) Effect of ocular pigmentation on hypotensive response to pilocarpine. *Am J Ophthalmol* **72**: 923–925.

47 Doughty MJ, Lyle WM (1991) Dapiprazole, an alpha adrenergic blocking drug, as an alternative miotic to pilocarpine or moxisylyte (thymoxamine) for reversing tropicamide mydriasis. *Can J Optom* **53**: 111–117.

48 Goldberg I, Ashburn FS, Kass MA *et al.* (1979) Efficacy and patient acceptance of pilocarpine gel. *Am J Ophthalmol* **88**: 843–846.

# Appendix – UK-marketed pharmaceuticals relevant to management of ocular diseases

**1.** *Eyelid cleansing products*

**Table 1   Eyelid cleansing products**

| drug name | conc. | C | PHARMACEUTICAL | corporate identification* | PRESENTATION |
|---|---|---|---|---|---|
| mixture of surfactants | n.a. | GSL | LID CARE (kit) | 1 | 80 ml bottle with pads |
| mixture of surfactants and cleansers | n.a. | GSL | LID CARE (sachets) | 1 | 20 pre-soaked sterile pads |

**2.** *Products for common hordeola (styes)*

**Table 2   Eyelid scrubs and select topical antibiotics for styes**

| drug name | conc. | C | PHARMACEUTICAL | corporate identification | PRESENTATION |
|---|---|---|---|---|---|
| lid scrubs | | | see Table 1 | | |
| dibromopropamidine | 0.15% | P | GOLDEN EYE | 2 | 3.5 g |
| | | P | BROLENE | 3 | 3.5 g |
| chloramphenicol | 0.5% | POM | CHLOROMYCETIN | 4 | 4 g |
| | | | CHLORAMPHENICOL | | 4 g |
| | | | CHLORAMPHENICOL (generics) | 5–11 | 4 g |

3. *Bacterial blepharoconjunctivitis essentially originating at and limited to the eyelid marginal zone*

**Table 3** **Eyelid scrubs, select topical antibiotics and mild corticosteroid ointments for bacterial blepharoconjunctivitis**

| drug name | conc. | C | PHARMACEUTICAL | corporate identification | PRESENTATION |
|---|---|---|---|---|---|
| chloramphenicol | 0.5% | POM | CHLOROMYCETIN CHLORAMPHENICOL (generics) | 4<br>5–11 | 4 g<br>4 g |
| polymyxin B with/bacitracin | 10000U 500U | POM | POLYFAX OPHTHALMIC OINTMENT | 14 | 4 g |
| polymyxin B with/trimethoprim | 10000U 0.1% | POM | POLYTRIM | 14 | 4 g |
| framycetin | 0.5% | POM | SOFRAMYCIN | 15 | 5 g |
| fusidic acid | 1.0% | POM | FUCITHALMIC | 16 | 5 g |
| chlortetracycline | 1.0% | POM | AUREOMYCIN | 17 | 3.5 g |
| hydrocortisone | 0.5% 1.0% 2.5% | POM | HYDROCORTISONE | 5 | 3 g |
| chloramphenicol w/ hydrocortisone | 0.5% 1.0% | POM | CHLOROMYCETIN H/C[a] | | 4 g |
| framycetin w/ dexamethasone plus gramicidin | 0.5% 0.6% 0.005% | POM | SOFRADEX | 15 | 5 g |
| hydrocortisone w/ nemoycin | 1.0% 0.5% | POM | NEO-CORTEF | 14 | 3.9 g |

[a] current availability uncertain as only a veterinary product is now listed (and not for human use)

## 4. *Bacterial conjunctivitis*

**Table 4** **Eyelid scrubs, topical antibiotics and topical mild corticosteroids for bacterial conjunctivitis**

| drug name | conc. | C | PHARMACEUTICAL | corporate identification | PRESENTATION |
|---|---|---|---|---|---|
| lid scrubs | | | see Table 1 | | |
| propamidine | 0.1% | P | GOLDEN EYE | 2 | 10 ml |
| | | P | BROLENE | 3 | 10 ml |
| chloramphenicol | 0.5% | POM | CHLOROMYCETIN | 4 | 5 or 10 ml |
| | | | SNO-PHENICOL | 18 | 10 ml |
| | | | CHLORAMPHENICOL | 5–13 | 10 ml |
| | | | MINIMS | | |
| | | | CHLORAMPHENICOL | 18 | unit dose |
| polymyxin B with/ trimethoprim | 10000U 0.1% | POM | POLYTRIM | 14 | 4 g |
| framycetin | 0.5% | POM | SOFRAMYCIN | 15 | 10 ml |
| gentamicin | 0.3% | POM | CIDOMYCIN[a] | 19 | 8 ml |
| | | | GARAMYCIN | 13 | 10 ml |
| | | | GENTICIN | 54 | |
| | | | MINIMS GENTAMICIN | 18 | unit dose |
| neomycin | 3500U 0.5% | POM | NEOMYCIN SULPHATE | 5 | 10 ml |
| | | | MINIMS NEOMYCIN | 18 | unit dose |
| fusidic acid (*gel*) | 1.0% | POM | FUCITHALMIC | 16 | 5 g |
| polymyxin B w/ trimethoprim | 10000U 0.1% | POM | POLYTRIM | 14 | 10 ml |
| polymyxin B w/ neomycin plus gramicidin | | POM | NEOSPORIN OPHTHALMIC SOLUTION | 14 | 5 ml |
| hydrocortisone w/ neomycin | 0.5% 0.5% | POM | NEO-CORTEF | 14 | 5 ml |
| clobetasone w/ neomycin | 0.1% 0.5% | POM | CLOBURATE-N | 14 | 10 ml |

[a] discontinued 7/2000

## 5. *Uncomplicated naso-lacrimal duct obstruction including mild dacryocystitis*

**Table 5    Topical ocular anaesthetics, fluorescein dye, sterile ophthalmic irrigants (eyewashes) and select topical antibiotics for naso-lacrimal duct obstruction**

| drug name | conc. | C | PHARMACEUTICAL | corporate identification | PRESENTATION |
|---|---|---|---|---|---|
| benoxinate | | POM | MINIMS BENOXINATE | 18 | unit dose |
| oxybuprocaine | | POM | MINIMS OXYBUPROCAINE | 18 | unit dose |
| fluorescein | 1% | POM | MINIMS FLUORESCEIN | 18 | unit dose |
| irrigating solution | | POM | IOCARE | 1 | 15 ml |
| chloramphenicol | 0.5% | POM | CHLOROMYCETIN | 4 | 5 or 10 ml |
| | | | SNO-PHENICOL | 18 | 10 ml |
| | | | CHLORAMPHENICOL (generic) | 5–13 | 10 ml |
| | | | MINIMS CHLORAMPHENICOL | 18 | unit dose |
| gentamicin | 0.3% | POM | MINIMS GENTAMICIN | 18 | unit dose |

## 6. *Non-infectious conjunctivitis caused by irritation*

**Table 6    Eyewashes, artificial tears, decongestants for non-infectious conjunctivitis caused by irritation**

| drug name | conc. | C | PHARMACEUTICAL | corporate identification | PRESENTATION |
|---|---|---|---|---|---|
| sodium chloride | 0.9% | P | NORMAL SALINE | 5 | 15 ml |
| | | | MINIMS SALINE | 18 | unit dose |
| witch hazel | 12% | GSL | OPTREX EYE LOTION | 20 | lotion 110 ml with eyecup |
| | | | VITAL EYES WASH | 1 | single use 10 ml ampoules |
| | | | I-DOC[a] | 21 | single use 10 ml ampoules |
| witch hazel | 12% | P | OPTREX EYEDROPS | 20 | 10 ml |
| witch hazel, glycerine | | P | OPTREX FRESH EYES | 20 | lotion 110 ml with eyecup |
| | | | OPTREX FRESH EYES Singles | 20 | unit dose |
| natural products | | SL | VITAL EYES | 1 | unit dose |
| | | | VITAL EYES MOISTURISER | 1 | 10 ml |
| | | GSL | VITAL EYES BRIGHTENER | 1 | 10 ml |
| | | GSL | RHOTO Zi for EYES | 21 | 8 ml |
| | | | EXTREME COOLING RHOTO Zi for EYES | 21 | 8 ml |
| | | SL | VIZULISE HERBAL EYE DROPS | 51 | 15 ml |
| phenylephrine | 0.12% | P | ISOPTO-FRIN | 22 | 10 ml |
| naphazoline | 0.012% | P | OPTREX CLEAR EYES | 20 | 10 ml |
| naphaloline | 0.012% | | MURINE | 23 | 10 ml |
| naphazoline | 0.012% | | EYE DEW CLEAR | 20 | 10 ml |
| naphazoline w/ brilliant blue | 0.012% | | EYE DEW BLUE | 20 | 10 ml |

[a] discontinued 8/1999

## 7. *Allergic conjunctivitis*

**Table 7    Saline, astringents, decongestants, topical antihistamines, mast cell stabilisers, oral antihistamines for chronic allergic conjunctivitis**

| drug name | conc. | C | PHARMACEUTICAL | corporate identification | PRESENTATION |
|---|---|---|---|---|---|
| saline and astringents | | | see Table 6 | | |
| decongestants | | | see Table 6 | | |
| antazoline with xylometazoline | 0.5% 0.05% | P | OTRIVIN-ANTISTIN | 1 | 10 ml |
| zinc sulphate | 0.25% | P | ZINC SULPHATE | 5 | 15 ml |
| levocabastine | 0.1% | P | LIVOSTIN DIRECT | 24 | 3 ml |
| levocabastine | 0.1% | POM | LIVOSTIN | 1 | 4 ml |
| azelastine | 0.05% | POM | OPTILAST | 25 | 4 ml |
| emedastine | | POM | EMADINE | 22 | |
| sodium cromoglycate | 2% | P | OPTICROM CLARITEYES HAY-CROM HAY FEVER RELIEF | 3 13 26 27 | 5 or 10 ml 10 ml 10 ml 10 ml |
| sodium cromoglycate | 2% | POM | OPTICROM HAY-CROM VIVIDRIN VIZ-ON SODIUM CROMOGLYCATE | 3 28 29 30 8,14,31 | 13.5 ml 13.5 ml 13.5 ml 13.5 ml 13.5 ml |
| lodoxamide | 0.1% | POM | ALOMIDE | 22 | 10 ml |
| nedocromil sodium | 2% | POM | RAPITIL | 3 | 5 ml |
| clobetasone | 0.1% | POM | CLOBURATE | 14 | 10 ml |
| fluorometholone | 0.1% | POM | FML | 32 | 5 ml |
| chlorpheniramine | 4 mg | P | PIRITON CALIMAL CHLORPHENIRAMINE (generic lines) | 33 34 6,8,35,36 | 4 mg × 30 4 mg × 30 4 mg × 30 |
| clemastine | | P/SL P | ALLER-EZE TAVEGIL | 39 40 | 1.34 mg × 10 or 30 1.35 mg × 60 |
| acrivastine | | P | BENADRYL ALLERGY RELIEF | 37 | 8 mg × 12 or 24 |
| loratidine | | P | CLARITYN | 13 | 10 mg × 7 |
| cetirizine | | P | ZIRTEK | 38 | 10 mg × 7 |
| cetirizine | | POM | ZIRTEK | 38 | 10 mg × 30 |

**8.** *Papillary conjunctivitis and contact lens-associated papillary conjunctivitis*

**Table 8  Topical mast cell stabilisers, topical mild corticosteroids for papillary and contact lens-associated papillary conjunctivitis, and select cases of follicular conjunctivitis**

| drug name | conc. | C | PHARMACEUTICAL | corporate identification | PRESENTATION |
|---|---|---|---|---|---|
| sodium cromoglycate | 2% | POM | OPTICROM | 3 | 13.5 ml |
| | | | HAY-CROM | 28 | 13.5 ml |
| | | | VIVIDRIN | 29 | 13.5 ml |
| | | | VIZ-ON | 30 | 13.5 ml |
| | | | SODIUM CROMOGLYCATE | 8, 14, 31 | 13.5 ml |
| lodoxamide | 0.1% | POM | ALOMIDE | 22 | 10 ml |
| nedocromil sodium | 2% | POM | RAPITIL | 3 | 5 ml |
| fluorometholone | 0.1% | POM | FML | 32 | 5 ml or 10 ml |
| betamethasone | 0.1% | POM | BETNESOL | 48 | 10 ml |
| | | | VISTA-METHASONE | 5 | 5 ml or 10 ml |

**9.** *Corneal inflammatory complications of contact lens wear including peripheral infiltrates*

**Table 9  Ocular lubricants and mild corticosteroids for corneal inflammatory complications of contact lens wear**

| drug name | conc. | C | PHARMACEUTICAL | corporate identification | PRESENTATION |
|---|---|---|---|---|---|
| ocular lubricants | | | see Table 10 | | |
| fluorometholone | 0.1% | POM | FML | 32 | 5 ml or 10 ml |
| betamethasone | 0.1% | POM | BETNESOL | 48 | 10 ml |
| | | | VISTA-METHASONE | 5 | 5 ml or 10 ml |

**10.** *Corneal foreign bodies and abrasions, and non-infectious superficial punctate keratitis*

**Table 10** **Topical antibiotic eyedrops, artificial tears and ocular lubricants for corneal foreign bodies and abrasions, and non-infectious superficial punctate keratitis**

| drug name | conc. | C | PHARMACEUTICAL | corporate identification | PRESENTATION |
|---|---|---|---|---|---|
| chloramphenicol | 0.5% | POM | MINIMS CHLORAMPHENICOL | 18 | unit dose |
| gentamicin | 0.3% | POM | MINIMS GENTAMICIN | 18 | unit dose |
| neomycin | 0.3% | | MINIMS NEOMYCIN | 18 | unit dose |
| polyvinyl alcohol | 1.4% | P | LIQUIFILM TEARS PF | 32 | unit dose |
| hypromellose | 0.5% | P | ARTELAC SDU | 29 | unit dose |
| hydroxyethylcellulose | 0.4% | P | MINIMS ARTIFICAL TEARS | 18 | unit dose |
| hydroxypropylmethylcellulose | 1.0% | P | ISOPTO ALKALINE | 22 | 15 ml |
| sodium hyaluronate | 0.18% | P | VISMED | 41 | unit dose |

**11.** *Ocular surface drying and discomfort associated with contact lens wear*

### Table 11   Contact lens wetting and rewetting solutions

| drug name | conc. | C | PHARMACEUTICAL | corporate identification* | PRESENTATION |
|---|---|---|---|---|---|
| sodium chloride c. hydroxypropylmethylcellulose and sorbic acid/EDTA | | CE | BAUSCH & LOMB RE-WETTING DROPS | 42 | 10 ml |
| sodium chloride c. hydroxyethylcellulose, poloxamer 406 and sorbic acid | | CE | CLERZ COMFORTING EYE DROPS | 1 | 10 ml |
| sodium chloride c. hydroxyethylcellulose, povidone, and polyhexanide/EDTA | | CE | OPTICIANS CHOICE COMFORT DROPS | 50 | 10 ml |
| sodium chloride c. polysorbate 80 and sodium citrate/EDTA | | CE | VIVA COMFORT DROPS[a] | 50 | 15 ml |
| sodium chloride and potassium, calcium and magnesium salts c. carboxymethylcellulose 0.5%, Purite | | SL | REFRESH CONTACTS | 32 | 15 ml |
| sodium chloride , dextran 70, hydroxypropylmethylcellulose, polidronium chloride, EDTA | | CE | OPTI-TEARS | 22 | 15 ml |
| sodium chloride c. hydroxyethylcellulose, poloxamer 406 | | CE | FOCUS CLERZ | 1 | unit dose |
| sodium chloride c. carboxymethylcellulose | | CE | REFRESH CONTACTS | 32 | unit dose |
| sodium chloride c. carboxymethylcellulose | | CE | REVIVE COMFORTING EYE DROPS | 32 | unit dose |
| hypromellose, sorbitol, EDTA | | P | ARTELAC SDU | 29 | unit dose |
| balanced salts mixture c. sodium hyaluronate | | P | VISMED LUBRICANT EYE DROPS | 41 | unit dose |
| balanced salts mixture c. sodium hyaluronate | | CE | VISLUBE | 53 | unit dose |
| sodium chloride, phosphate buffer, hyalan fluid 0.15% | | CE | i.com COMFORT SHIELD | 52 | unit dose |
| sodium chloride c. PEG 300 BP, and polyoxyl 40 stearate | | CE | LENS FRESH COMFORT AND RE-WETTING DROPS[b] | 32 | unit dose |

[a] product imported into UK   [b] discontinued 1999

**12.** *Superficial non-infectious corneal epithelial disease to include dry eye and recurrent corneal erosion*

**Table 12    Artificial tears, ocular lubricants, and mucolytic agents for superficial non-infectious corneal epithelial disease to include dry eye and recurrent corneal erosion**

| drug name | conc. | C | PHARMACEUTICAL | corporate identification | PRESENTATION |
|---|---|---|---|---|---|
| hypromellose | 0.3% | P | MOISTURE TEARS | 7 | 10 ml |
|  | 0.3% | P | EYEDROPS | 27 | 10 ml |
|  | 0.3% | GSL | OPTREX DRY EYE THERAPY[a] | 20 |  |
|  | 0.4% | P | HYPROMELLOSE (generic) | 5, 6, 8 9–11, 13 | 10 ml |
|  | 0.5% | P | ISOPTO PLAIN | 22 | 10 ml |
| hypromellose | 0.5% | P | ARTELAC SDU | 29 | unit dose |
| hypromellose c. dextran 70 | 0.3% 0.1% | P | TEARS NATURALE | 1 | 15 ml |
| polyvinyl alcohol | 1.4% | P | LIQUIFILM TEARS | 32 | 15 ml |
|  | 1.4% |  | SNO TEARS | 18 | 10 ml |
|  | 1.0% |  | HYPOTEARS | 1 | 10 ml |
| polyvinyl alcohol | 1.4% | P | LIQUIFILM TEARS PF | 32 | unit dose |
| polyvinyl alcohol c. povidone | 1.4% 0.6% | P | REFRESH | 32 | unit dose |
| sodium chloride EDTA hyproxyethylcellulose polixetonium chloride | 0.1% 0.36% 0.006% | SL | REFRESH INSTANT REVIVAL EYE DROPS | 32 | 15 ml |
| sodium chloride, carboxymethylcellulose | 0.5% | SL | REFRESH SOOTHE AND PROTECT EYE DROPS | 32 | unit dose |
| polyvidone | 5.0% | P | OCULOTECT | 1 | unit dose |
| hydroxypropylmethylcellulose | 1.0% | P | ISOPTO ALKALINE | 22 | 15 ml |
| sodium hyaluronate | 0.18% | P | VISMED | 41 | unit dose |
| carbomer 940 | 0.2% | P | VISCOTEARS | 1 | 5 g |
|  | 0.2% | P | GELTEARS | 18 | 5 g or 10 g |
| white paraffin |  | P | LUBRI-TEARS | 22 | 5 g |
|  |  | P | LACRI-LUBE | 32 | 3.5 g or 5 g |
| yellow paraffin |  | P | SIMPLE EYE OINTMENT | 5 | 4 g |
| acetylcysteine c. hypromellose | 5% 0.3% | POM | ILUBE | 32 | 10 ml |

[a] discontinued 2/1998

## 13. *Superficial herpes viral diseases of the conjunctiva and cornea*

**Table 13   Topical anti-viral drugs for superficial herpes viral diseases of the conjunctiva and cornea**

| drug name | conc. | C | PHARMACEUTICAL | corporate identification | PRESENTATION |
|-----------|-------|---|----------------|--------------------------|--------------|
| acyclovir | 3% | POM | ZOVIRAX | 43 | 4.5 g |

## 14. *Superficial adenoviral or enteroviral diseases of the conjunctiva and cornea*

**Table 14   Topical anti-viral drug, decongestants, mild corticosteroids for superficial adenoviral-type diseases of the conjunctiva and cornea**

| drug name | conc. | C | PHARMACEUTICAL | corporate identification | PRESENTATION |
|-----------|-------|---|----------------|--------------------------|--------------|
| decongestants | | | see Table 6 | | |
| acyclovir | 3% | POM | ZOVIRAX | 43 | 4.5 g |
| hydrocortisone | 0.5% 1.0% 2.5% | POM | HYDROCORTISONE (generic) | | |
| clobetasone | 0.1% | POM | CLOBURATE | 14 | 10 ml |
| fluorometholone | 0.1% | POM | FML | 32 | 5 ml |
| betamethasone | 0.1% | POM | BETNESOL VISTA-METHASONE | 48 5 | 10 ml 5 ml or 10 ml |

## 15. *Mild corneal and anterior segment inflammatory disease*

**Table 15   Mild corticosteroids, cycloplegics for mild corneal and anterior segment inflammatory disease**

| drug name | conc. | C | PHARMACEUTICAL | corporate identification | PRESENTATION |
|-----------|-------|---|----------------|--------------------------|--------------|
| atropine | 1.0% 0.5% 1.0% | POM | ISPTO ATROPINE ATROPINE ATROPINE (generic) | 22 5 5, 13 | 5 ml 10 ml 10 ml |
| homatropine | 1% 2% 2% | POM | HOMATROPINE HOMATROPINE ISOPTO HOMATROPINE[a] | 5 5 22 | 10 ml 10 ml 15 ml |
| atropine | 1.0% | POM | ATROPINE | 5 | 3 g |
| clobetasone | 0.1% | POM | CLOBURATE | 14 | 10 ml |
| fluorometholone | 0.1% | POM | FML | 32 | 5 ml |
| betamethasone | 0.1% | POM | BETNESOL VISTA-METHASONE | 48 5 | 10 ml 5 ml or 10 ml |

[a] current availability uncertain

**16.** *Anti-inflammatory drugs for moderate-to-severe inflammatory disease, including post-operative care*

**Table 16  Strong-to-potent corticosteroids for uveal inflammations and post-operative care of inflammation**

| drug name | conc. | C | PHARMACEUTICAL | corporate identification | PRESENTATION |
|---|---|---|---|---|---|
| fluorometholone | 0.1% | POM | FML | 32 | 5 ml |
| betamethasone | 0.1% | POM | BETNESOL | 48 | 10 ml |
| | | | VISTA-METHASONE | 5 | 5 ml or 10 ml |
| dexamethasone | 0.1% | POM | MINIMS DEXAMETHASONE | 18 | unit dose |
| | | | MAXIDEX | 22 | 5 ml or 10 ml |
| prednisolone | 0.5% | POM | MINIMS PREDNISOLONE | 18 | unit dose |
| | | | PREDSOL | 48 | 10 ml |
| prednisolone | 1.0% | POM | PRED FORTE | | 5 ml or 10 ml |
| rimexolone | 1.0% | POM | VEXOL | 22 | 5 ml |

**17.** *Moderate-to-severe bacterial infections of the cornea and conjunctiva*

**Table 17  Broad spectrum antibacterial drugs for moderate-to-severe severe bacterial conjunctivitis, bacterial keratitis and bacterial ulcers of the cornea**

| drug name | conc. | C | PHARMACEUTICAL | corporate identification | PRESENTATION |
|---|---|---|---|---|---|
| ciprofloxacin | 0.3% | POM | CILOXAN | 22 | 5 ml |
| ofloxacin | 0.3% | POM | EXOCIN | 32 | 5 ml |
| lomefloxacin | 0.3% | POM | OKACYN | 1 | 5 ml |

**18.** *Coordinated-care of angle-closure glaucoma*

**Table 18  Oral ocular hypotensive drugs and miotics for coordinated care of angle-closure glaucoma**

| drug name | conc. | C | PHARMACEUTICAL | corporate identification | PRESENTATION |
|---|---|---|---|---|---|
| acetazolamide | | POM | DIAMOX | 17 | 250 mg tab |
| | | POM | ACETAZOLAMIDE | 44 | 250 mg tab |
| glycerin | | GSL | GLYCERINE (GLYCEROL) | | 110 ml (6 oz measure = 1 dose) |
| pilocarpine | 2 or 4% | POM | MINIMS PILO | 18 | unit dose |
| | 2 or 4% | POM | ISOPTO CARPINE | 1 | 10 ml |
| | 2 or 4% | POM | SNO-CARPINE[a] | 18 | 10 ml |
| | 2 or 4% | POM | PILOCARPINE | 5, 8, 9, 11, 13 | 10 ml |

[a] discontinued 8/1999

## 19. *Shared-care of primary open-angle glaucoma*

**Table 19  Ocular hypotensive agents for coordinated care of open-angle glaucoma, ocular hypertension and normal tension glaucoma**

| drug name | conc. | C | PHARMACEUTICAL | corporate identification | PRESENTATION |
|---|---|---|---|---|---|
| timolol | 0.25% | POM | TIMOPTOL | 45 | 5 ml |
| | 0.25% | | GLAU-OPT | 30 | 5 ml |
| | 0.25% | | TIMOLOL (generic) | 1, 6, 8, 9, 12, 31, 47 | 5 ml |
| | 0.5% | | TIMOPTOL | 54 | 5 ml |
| | 0.5% | | GLAU-OPT | 30 | 5 ml |
| | 0.5% | | TIMOLOL (g) | 1, 6, 8, 9, 12, 31, 47 | 5 ml |
| timolol | 0.25% | | TIMOLOL LA | 45 | 2.5 ml |
| | 0.5% | | | | |
| levobunolol | 0.5% | POM | BETAGAN | 32 | 5 ml |
| | 0.5% | | BETAGAN UNIT DOSE | 32 | unit dose |
| | | | LEVOBUNOLOL (generic)[a] | | 5 ml |
| betaxolol | 0.25% | POM | BETOPTIC SUSPENSION | 22 | 5ml |
| betaxolol | 0.5% | POM | BETOPTIC DROPS | 22 | 5 ml |
| carteolol | 1% | POM | TEOPTIC | 1 | 10 ml |
| | 2% | | | | 10 ml |
| adrenaline (epinephrine) | 1% | POM | SIMPLENE | 18 | 7.5 ml |
| | 2% | | SIMPLENE | | 7.5 ml |
| dipivefrin | 0.1% | POM | PROPINE | 32 | 5 ml or 10 ml |
| | | | DIPIVEFRINE (generic) | 22 | 10 ml |
| brimonidine | 0.2% | POM | ALPHAGAN | 32 | 5 ml |
| guanethidine c. | 1/0.2 | POM | GANDA | 18 | 7.5 ml |
| adrenaline (epinephrine) | 3/0.5 | | GANADA | | 7.5 ml |
| dorzolamide | 2% | POM | TRUSOPT | 45 | 5 ml |
| brinzolamide | 1% | POM | AZOPT | 22 | 5 ml or 10 ml |
| dorzolamide c. | 2% | POM | COSOPT | 45 | 5 ml |
| timolol | 0.5% | | | | |
| latanoprost | 0.02% | POM | XALATAN | 49 | 2.5 ml |
| pilocarpine | 2.0% | POM | ISOPTO CARPINE | 22 | 10 ml |
| | 2.0% | | SNO-CARPINE[b] | 18 | 10 ml |
| | 2.0% | | PILOCARPINE (generic) | 5, 8, 9, 11, 13 | 10 ml |
| | 3.0% | | ISOPTO CARPINE | 22 | 10 ml |
| | 3.0% | | SNO-CARPINE[b] | 18 | 10 ml |
| | 3.0% | | PILOCARPINE (generic) | 5, 8, 9, 11, 13 | 10 ml |
| | 4.0% | | ISOPTO CARPINE | 22 | 10 ml |
| | 4.0% | | SNO-CARPINE[b] | 18 | 10 ml |
| | 4.0% | | PILOCARPINE (generic) | 5, 8, 9, 11, 13 | 10 ml |
| pilocarpine | 4.0% | POM | PILOGEL | 22 | 5 g |
| pilocarpine | 20 mcg | POM | OCUSERT P-20 | 14 | ophthalmic insert |
| | 40 mcg | | OCUSERT P-40 | | pkg 2 |
| carbachol | 1.5% | POM | ISOPTO CARBACHOL | 22 | 15 ml |
| | 3.0% | | ISOPTO CARBACHOL | | 15 ml |

[a] current availability uncertain but products have been marketed  [b] discontinued 8/1999

CORPORATE IDENTIFICATION KEY FOR TABLES

**1.** Ciba Vision Ophthalmics, **2.** Typharm, **3.** Rhone-Poulenc-Rorer, **4.** Forley, **5.** Martindale, **6.** APS, **7.** C-Pharma, **8.** Cox Pharms, **9.** Hillcross Pharms, **10.** Norton Healthcare, **11.** Stevenden Healthcare, **12.** Cusi, **13.** Schering-Plough, **14.** Dominion, **15.** Florizel (Distriphar), **16.** Leo Pharms, **17.** Wyeth Labs, **18.** Chauvin, **19.** Hoechst-Marion Roussel, **20.** Crookes Healthcare, **21.** Metholatum, **22.** Alcon, **23.** Abbott, **24.** Johnson & Johnson, **25.** ASTA Medical, **26.** Norton Consumer, **27.** Boots, **28.** Baker Norton Pharms, **29.** NuCare, **30.** Opus Pharms, **31.** Genus Pharms, **32.** Allergan, **33.** Stafford-Miller, **34.** Sussex Pharms, **35.** Cross-Pharma, **36.** NuMark, **37.** Warner Lambert Consumer, **38.** UCB Pharma, **39.** Novartis Consumer Health, **40.** Novartis Pharms, **41.** Surgical Designs, **42.** Bausch & Lomb Surgical, **43.** Wellcome, **44.** Regent Labs, **45.** Merck Sharpe & Dohme, **46.** Bioglan, **47.** Generics UK, **48.** Medeva-Pharma, **49.** Pharmacia & Upjohn, **50.** Nissel, **51.** Peach Pharma, **52.** Chrome-x, **53.** Chemedica, **54.** Roche.

# Index

# Subscribe to Optician

## And receive your own personal copy every week

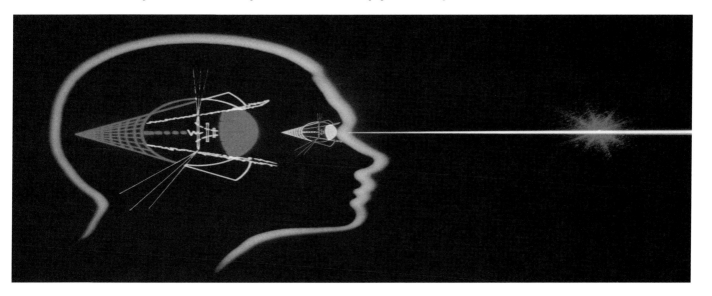

- exclusive news coverage
- latest job vacancies
- fashion trends
- approved continuing education
- college approved CET
- clinical and technical features

- business management information
  AND a range of supplements throughout the year:
- eyestyle
- instrument insight
- optical technician
- recruitment
- optical yearbook
- wallplanner

For current subscription rates simply telephone 01444 475634 or fax 01444 445447
Quote code 124.

Or fill in the coupon below and return it to: Optician Subscriptions, FREEPOST RCC2619, HAYWARDS HEATH,
RH16 3BR
(please affix stamp if posted outside the UK)

---

## Optician

☐ **Please send me the current subscription rates for Optician**

Title          Initial          Surname _____

Job title _____

Address     ☐ home     ☐ practice _____

_____

Postcode _____     Telephone _____          Code 124

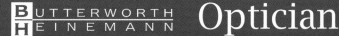